AGRICULTURE

POCKET LIBRARY OF SPIRITUAL WISDOM

Practical Applications

Also in this series:

(Practical Applications)
Architecture
Art
Education
Medicine
Religion
Science
Social and Political Science

(Esoteric)
Alchemy
Atlantis
Christian Rozenkreutz
The Druids
The Goddess
The Holy Grail

RUDOLF STEINER

AGRICULTURE
An Introductory Reader

*Compiled with an introduction,
commentary and notes by
Richard Thornton Smith*

Sophia Books

All translations revised by Christian von Arnim

Sophia Books
An imprint of Rudolf Steiner Press
Hillside House, The Square
Forest Row, RH18 5ES

www.rudolfsteinerpress.com

Published by Rudolf Steiner Press 2003

For earlier English publications of individual selections please
see pp. 225–30

The material by Rudolf Steiner was originally published in
German in various volumes of the 'GA' (*Rudolf Steiner
Gesamtausgabe* or Collected Works) by Rudolf Steiner Verlag,
Dornach. This authorized volume is published by permission of
the Rudolf Steiner Nachlassverwaltung, Dornach (for further
information see pp. 235–6)

A catalogue record for this book is available from the British
Library

ISBN 1 85584 113 4

Cover by Andrew Morgan Design
Typeset by DP Photosetting, Aylesbury, Bucks.
Printed and bound in Great Britain by Cromwell Press Limited,
Trowbridge, Wilts.

Contents

Introduction

by Richard Thornton Smith

The current context of agriculture

Most of us would probably agree that the mission of agriculture is to feed humanity. This book of extracts from Rudolf Steiner's works explores the breadth and depth of meaning in this statement. But before offering an outline of the book it is necessary to make a few observations about people and agriculture so as to place the material in a truly modern context.

Agriculture was once a way of life connecting human beings with the earth and her rhythms, but this relationship has been progressively eroded by an urbanizing world driven by commercial imperatives. It is true that mechanization has emancipated us from the toils inflicted on Adam, while the starvation visualized by Malthus has up to now been localized and linked to conflict and poverty as much as environment. On the other hand, society — Western society in particular — has massive social and mental health problems. The latter may well be partly linked to the nutritional quality of our food, now heavily compromised by farming and food processing methods.[1] Many problems can be seen as resulting from the dominance of economic forces over other aspects of human life. In agriculture we see the human consequences both of driving down food prices and of advancing technology and chemicals. The current health and safety risks in agriculture together with the terrible consequences of bankruptcy now make farming one of the highest-risk occupations in the world.

In this modern world all human activities are driven by and subordinated to economic processes, whether local or global. The environmental and social consequences of this are now outstandingly obvious in developed and developing countries alike.

Farming is part of the culture of every land and it has been fundamental to civilization in providing the foundation from which a variety of economic activities have developed. As the world becomes ever more dependent upon non-agricultural work, it becomes increasingly important to realize this. Such an urban orientation has already shaped the public and political attitude to agriculture. Instead of being able to follow its own rules dictated by natural processes and local markets, agriculture has become a slave to a distant majority who have little knowledge of its inner workings and who find it natural to regard a farm as being like any other production system.[2] It is sobering to reflect that as world population increases, total food production is in the hands of a dwindling number of farm workers whose daily tasks and financial rewards would be considered unacceptable by the majority. It is even claimed that young people today are no longer capable of the physical work required.

In recent years the public have been faced with a variety of scares ranging from the pesticide content of vegetables to the consequences of feeding cattle with animal waste products. These events are welcome in the sense that they have provided a wake-up call. The recent period of chemical agriculture and food processing has seen unprecedented increases in the incidence of certain diseases and it may yet have such an influence upon human fertility that no other population control measure will have been as successful. Increased awareness has been a turning-point in food budgeting for many people, yet the current low food price culture and the seductive influence of junk foods is a huge obstacle to a healthier society. The food industry together with the majority of consumers consider that the way we produce our food doesn't matter, that carbohydrate or protein is the same however it is produced or reconstituted. At a time when health service provision is constantly in the spotlight it might seem difficult to comprehend why there are no hard-hitting national initiatives to build positive health through diet and nutrition. Were the truth to be known, understood and adequately researched, the situation could be so different. As it is, even those inclining towards organic produce do so for reasons which are mostly peripheral to an understanding of its real health benefits.

Background to the present volume

This clearly identifies an objective towards which a deeper knowledge of agriculture and human needs should be directed. It is no use blaming a system that is profoundly ignorant of the human being and our connection with the wide realms of nature. The rebuilding of a knowledge that people once had, but transformed through the modern intellect and expressed through our independent life-styles, will in the future enable us to change the market-place and to refashion the world. Rudolf Steiner devoted his life's energies to further our spiritual understanding of the human being, and his work is alive with relevance to the situation we face at the present time. He addressed himself to the many subjects with a bearing on natural science or agriculture, however remote some of these topics might appear. Indeed, in his agriculture lectures we read that 'there is scarcely a realm of human life which lies outside our subject'. Throughout the preparation of this book I have had in mind Steiner's reply to a question put to him by Ehrenfried Pfeiffer concerning people's lack of will and progress with spiritual activities despite his stimulus and guidance. Steiner answered, 'This is a problem of nutrition. Nutrition as it is today does not supply the strength necessary for manifesting the spirit in physical life. A bridge can no longer be built from thinking to will and action. Food plants no longer contain the forces people need for this.'[3]

Steiner grew up in a landscape where traditional

knowledge was still alive, so he understood much about the nature of farming. Yet it was only in the last year of his life, and then after intensive persuasion, that he finally gave the course of lectures which set new horizons for how we should view and practise agriculture. The problems which were arising at that time and on which Steiner was urged to speak would seem familiar today, namely, a decline of soil fertility, seed vitality and animal health.[4] But Steiner also stated ominously that there might come a time when we would be unable to grow our crops because the earth's natural vitality was in decline. The means to averting this problem lies with humankind, providing we are willing to adopt appropriate attitudes and measures.

It should be pointed out that in Steiner's day most of the larger farms were already employing chemical fertilizers while organic-ecological farming in the modern sense was not recognized, still less established. It was to the owners of large commercial farms as well as to those familiar with Steiner's spiritual science that the agriculture lectures were addressed. Thus, even in purely organic farming terms Rudolf Steiner ranks as a pioneer and visionary.[5] Those meeting this material for the first time should realize that Steiner did not invent any special name with which to identify his agricultural message. That fell to those who began to research his suggestions in a practical way.[6] Thus the appellation *biodynamic agriculture* arose — implying a connection with living energies.

Although agriculture is pre-eminently a practical activity to which Steiner offered his own practical ideas, his contribution is best characterized as providing a background to understanding agriculture so that it might develop creatively in the future. Nowhere does he proclaim that the modern scientific outlook and the facts which it discovers are incorrect, rather that they are one-sided and represent the corpse of the physical realm rather than its living reality. He is, above all, concerned to inform us about what lies behind the visible part of natural science. Thus we learn that all life is dependent on form and life-giving energies received from the cosmos, from sun and starry constellations, from moon and planets. We learn, too, of how our soil can be made more sensitive to receive these energies and to transmit them to the growth of plants. Such deep wisdom is clearly not 'lesson one' in agriculture but is aimed at raising the awareness of those already familiar with farming practices. Steiner thus guides us in a new way of working with the forces of nature which, once understood, can profoundly affect the attitude of the farmer or gardener to their work.

The *Agriculture Course* inevitably provides much material for the present volume. Like most of Steiner's works it requires repeated study in order to gain a good foothold and it is essential to be open to Steiner's other major works in order to progress with it.[7] Be assured, however, of eventual rewards. Steiner himself said that 'the best books are those we have to take up again and again, books we cannot understand immediately but have to study sentence by sentence'.[8]

Overview of contents

The book has been divided into ten chapters, which allow the exploration of a broad range of material from the esoteric to the more obviously practical. In view of the unique nature of the book's subject matter it was decided to allow the first and last chapters to provide a framework from a spiritual perspective. These chapters, though they touch on agriculture and nutrition, thus mainly provide the intervening chapters with a foundation and a logical conclusion. The overall sequence forms a kind of journey.

We start by looking back at history and consider the cosmic sources upon which our existence depends. We proceed to examine aspects of our farm work and end up looking at the importance of a balanced working of these influences for our health and the future tasks of humanity. The reader will realize that any anthology reflects both the personal choice and limits of knowledge of the editor and what might appear as a balanced picture to some will surely not satisfy others. The task of creating a tree out of prunings is certainly not an easy one. I am conscious that short extracts may violate the integrity of the original and risk creating a fragmented text. However, the aim has been to draw widely from available material and thereby open windows onto more of Steiner's works.

In Chapter 1 we begin with the constitution of the human being and then look back at former conditions of Earth, which the human being experienced while not yet in a solid material condition. Human consciousness has evolved with the physical and it would certainly be salutary for historians and archaeologists to be aware that the faculty of logical thinking is a recent acquisition for the great mass of humanity. The history of nutrition not surprisingly parallels this course. We did not need food in the contemporary sense until our physical bodies had densified from the surrounding ether; this occurred during Atlantean times (the late Tertiary period), before our present epoch. Knowledge of our spiritual origins certainly helps us understand the remarks Steiner makes concerning the cosmic aspect of nutrition at the present time. We also learn about the role or mission of certain foods and drink in the course of our evolution. It is clear that in some cases these materials have little further use unless our spiritual path is to be impeded.

Chapter 2 looks outward to sun and stars — to the source of etheric energy on which life here depends. The living nature of what astronomy simply regards as point sources of light has to be grasped, as also does the concept of the sun as a suctional hollow sphere gathering the forces coming from the wider periphery of stars and raying these out across the solar system. The four essential elements of life — earth, water, air and warmth — were recognized by ancient people across the world. Spiritual essences of these elements — ethers — were known to arise from the different constellations of what came to be known as the zodiac. When sun or moon lie in front of particular constellations their character changes as the influence of each constellation is blocked. This causes the plant being to strive harder to compensate for the temporary imbalance in cosmic forces. Biodynamics makes use of this principle to select the most appropriate times for agricultural tasks.

Chapter 3 takes a closer look at the plant world. Looking at earth history it is noted that all matter — even our solid rock formations — has passed through a plantlike and therefore living condition. We are made aware of the plant as a vital link between the living earth and the spiritual beings of the sun. Moreover, each part of the earth experiences a diurnal and annual breathing process with plant life playing an essential part in this rhythmic activity. This seasonal rhythm is employed in the preparation of particular substances for biodynamic agriculture. The astrality or consciousness of the cosmos which envelops plants, especially strong in the case of trees, is of the greatest benefit to the earth's fertility. In this connection the existence of birds and insects — the honey bee in particular — is of vital importance. We therefore understand from a new vantage point how increasingly disastrous it will become for the earth's agricultural capabilities as further biodiversity is lost and as forest cover diminishes.

In Chapter 4 we see that the ideal farm should also be a reflection of the whole spiritual organism of the earth. The ideal of an organic-ecological farm functioning like an organism with products from one activity contributing raw materials to another is now widely acknowledged. The farm animal, notably the cow, consumes the plant and through concentrating forces within its digestive system returns vitality to the earth through its dung. This has a special significance for the place where the animals grazed, so it is possible to understand why importation of fertility onto a farm is far from ideal. Meanwhile birds and insects not only spread beneficent influences to the plant world but return an image of material existence to beings in the spiritual world. This and the importance of preserving habitats for all forms of wildlife, fungi included, underlines the fact that if we allow nature her place our best interests will be served.

Chapter 5 must surely alter our view of chemical substances. A view of the atom as a bubble associated with matter and force was surely controversial in its time but is largely supportive of the vision of earlier occultists. We then hear how contrasting planetary influences connect in the earth with silica and lime substances to create a balanced foundation for life processes. There are the forces which support the outward display of growth and reproductive activity while others infuse substance with energy and act more qualitatively to create colour and other sensory characteristics. Chemical farming supports pre-eminently the former type of growth, and hence certain essential aspects of food quality are deficient. In the final section Steiner explains the spiritual tasks of each of the main elements of organic matter. Taken collectively this is a story that points to the primacy of the spiritual world and the impermanence of materiality.

Those aware of organic farming principles will realize the importance of organic matter in supporting soil life and humus content. The question for Chapter 6 is: can we begin to understand how it is from a supersensible point of view? We are told that forces coming from the outer planets must penetrate earthly substance otherwise growth will be unbalanced. To accomplish this, a living soil is needed to generate humus. This then forms close associations with clay, linking the organic and purely mineral worlds. Steiner shows, too, that there is more to a compost pile than decomposition and that minor elements are rayed into the soil from the cosmos in a healthy organic soil. Later in the chapter we are confronted by the most profound of life's processes — the relationship between cosmic life forces and the inspiration of the 'universal all' of cosmic space or chaos. Here too, we see how crucial are conditions within the soil for the proper interplay of these activities.

Chapter 7 concentrates on special measures which Steiner indicated could be employed to support the working of cosmic forces within soil and plant. It is because the earth's vitality is steadily declining — no doubt worsened in recent times — that instructions for making particular materials were left to us. The implication behind these vitalizing biodynamic preparations, each of which has particular planetary relationships, is that organic methods alone may in a future time be insufficient to promote productive growth. The methods recommended for weed and pest problems, designed to bring about a natural balance rather than eradicate the organism, negatively affect reproduction and utilize specific cosmic timings.

In Chapter 8 we encounter the elemental beings, about which Steiner spoke on many occasions, though only one brief reference is made to them in the *Agriculture Course*. One group of these have a special connection to the growth of plants. They are the animating forces behind otherwise inanimate processes such as plant nutrient uptake or photosynthesis. Although we cannot see them they can perceive our thoughts and feelings. At present this realm of beings needs our conscious support.[9]

Chapter 9 examines human and animal nutrition. We have ultimately to understand that nutrition involves two streams, one earthly — about which we think we know a great deal — and one cosmic. The earthly stream rises to meet the cosmic in the body. Fine cosmic influences enter us through our breathing and through our different sense organs. The forces from our food enter the different parts of our body to facilitate this process. The cosmic thus takes hold of life energies to create our bodily substance. These energies are especially promoted through organic and biodynamic husbandry. Steiner indicates that the effects of a healthy nutrition are even more evident in subsequent generations, a fact borne out by recent research.

Chapter 10 considers a few aspects of our work in shaping the future. Steiner made it clear on many occasions that it is humanity's task in the future to raise itself and to spiritualize the earth. We are urged to develop our inner spiritual qualities, to direct our energies towards helping others and becoming aware of the needs of other spiritual beings for our help and for our moral actions —

such actions affecting our environment in ways previously unsuspected. We must also develop a special personal relationship with what we do. For most of us the first step in this is to be sufficiently conscious of the present moment and not always be thinking of what we have to do next! As human beings develop higher faculties this personal factor is destined to bring results in the field of nature more effectively than in any other way. But to accomplish a great deal of this we need the right nutrition to support our spiritual striving and to generate appropriate forces of will. Nutrition is emphasized in these pages precisely because it has to play such a crucial role in our further evolution. Forces that stand in the way of a better nutrition must be clearly identified as opposing the true path of humankind.

To end, I should like to acknowledge all those who, through discussion and practical experience have helped me over recent years to draw nearer to involvement in and understanding of biodynamic work. These include especially Jimmy and Pauline Anderson, Alan Brockman, Matthias Guépin, Bernard Jarman, Hans-Günther Kern, Walter Rudert, Freya Schikorr and Patricia Thompson. I also thank Rainer Bauer, Joan Brinch, Timothy Brink, David Clement and Tyll van de Voort for comments and information while working on this volume. Thanks are also due to Margaret Jonas, Librarian at Rudolf Steiner House, and to Sevak Gulbekian of Rudolf Steiner Press.

1. The Evolving Human Being

Rudolf Steiner indicates that the history of our part of the universe — our solar system — is inextricably linked to the creation and progress of humanity. This humanity has 'condensed' from spiritual realms and now fully manifests on the physical plane in a way never previously experienced by humankind nor even by those spiritual powers which have guided the evolutionary process. In this first chapter we learn of the different elements of our human being before considering our former states of existence. In this respect we should realize that former incarnations (or planetary conditions) of the earth — frequently spoken of in Steiner's works — have been vehicles for the progressive construction of the human being, initially undifferentiated but now experienced in a female or male aspect. At each stage of this long evolution, human beings have cast off coarser elements of their nature and substance in order to advance spiritually. These laid-aside elements are the other kingdoms of nature: the mineral, plant and animal. This, of course, is quite the reverse picture of evolution to what has become accepted in the last two centuries.

The current earth stage of evolution is the fourth major episode in human development, of which there will be seven. Each major period is divided into seven stages and each of these into seven smaller ones, making a total of 343. Time itself is not to be thought of as linear. Instead, what we experience as time today, bound by our physical bodies, is much more prolonged than it has been or

*will be in the future. It is not until well into the earth stage of our
evolution that we can properly trace an emergence of the consciousness we experience today. The acquisition of a modern sense
of identity and intellectual capability has only occurred more
generally within the last 500 years. As new faculties have
emerged, earlier ones have been lost. In parallel with such
development and perhaps accelerating it, changes in nutrition
have occurred. Such changes not only make us think about the
significance of the different diets people experience across the
world but highlight the importance of an awareness of diet and
nutrition in assisting our advancement as human beings.*

The contemporary human being

Let us first consider the nature and essence of the human
being. When someone comes into our presence, we first of
all see the physical body through our sense organs. The
human being has this body in common with the whole
world around him; and although the physical body is only
a small part of what the human being really is, it is the
only part of which ordinary science takes account. But we
must go deeper. Human beings can move, feel and think;
they grow, take nourishment and reproduce their kind.
Human beings have in common with plants their capacity
to nourish themselves, to grow and reproduce; if they
were like stones, with only a physical body, none of this
would be possible. They must therefore possess something which enables them to use substances and their

forces in such a way that they become for them the means of growth. This is the etheric body.[10]

The human being, of course, has other faculties as well. He can feel pleasure and pain, which the plant cannot do. Animals can feel pleasure and pain, and thus have a further principle in common with the human being: the astral body.[11] The astral body is the seat of everything we know as desire, passion, and so forth.

But the human being is distinguished from the animal. This brings us to the fourth element of the human being which comes to expression in a name different from all other names. I can say 'I' only of myself.[12] The higher the moral and intellectual development of a human being, the more will his 'I' have worked upon the astral body.

Whatever part of the astral body has been thus transformed by the 'I' is called Manas. Manas is the fifth member of the human being's nature. A human being has just so much of Manas as he has created by his own efforts; part of his astral body is therefore always Manas. But the human being is not able to exercise an immediate influence upon the etheric body, although in the same way that he can raise himself to a higher moral level he can also learn to work upon the etheric body. What he has transformed in this body by his own efforts is called Buddhi. This is the sixth element of the human being's nature.

The highest achievement open to the human being is to work right down into his physical body. That is the most difficult task of all. In order to have an effect upon the physical body, the human being must learn to control the breath and the circulation, to follow consciously the activity of the nerves, and to regulate the processes of thought.[13] He will then have developed in himself what we call Atma. In every human being four elements are fully formed, the fifth only partly, the sixth and seventh only in rudimentary form. Physical body, etheric body, astral body, 'I' or ego, Manas, Buddhi, Atma—these are the seven constituent elements of the human being.

Former evolutionary stages

As an individual, the human being has to pass through different stages after birth. Just as he must ascend from infancy through childhood and so on to the age of the mature adult, so too must humankind as a whole go through a similar process. Humanity has developed to its present condition by passing through other stages. With the methods of the clairvoyant one can discern three principal stages of such development of humankind, which were passed through before the formation of the earth took place. At present we are concerned with the fourth stage in the great universal life of the human being.

The human being existed before there was an earth. But one must not imagine that he had previously lived on other planets and then at a certain time migrated to earth. Rather, Earth has developed together with the human being. Earth has passed through three main stages of development before becoming what we now call the 'earth'. We must completely liberate ourselves from the meaning that contemporary science associates with the names 'Saturn', 'Sun' and 'Moon' if we want to understand the explanations of the scientist of the spirit.

Before the heavenly body on which the life of the human being takes place became 'earth', it was Moon, before that Sun, and yet earlier Saturn. One can assume three further principal stages which Earth still has to pass through — these have been named Jupiter, Venus and Vulcan. Thus the heavenly body with which human destiny is connected has passed through three stages in the past, is now in its fourth, and will in the future have to pass through three more until all the talents which the human being has within himself are developed, until he arrives at the peak of his perfection.

During the Saturn stage of Earth evolution, only the first germs of the kingdom of the human being dwelt on it. The marvellously artistic structure of the human body was then present only in barest outline. There were no minerals, plants or animals. The human being is the first-born of our creative process. But the human being on Saturn was very different from the human being of today. He was for the most part a spiritual being; he would not have been visible to physical eyes.

Now just as the human being passes through the various stages of his life — as child, young man or woman, old man or woman — so does a planet. Before Saturn manifested the flaky structures deposited within it, it was an Arupa-Devachan structure, then a Rupa-Devachan structure, and finally an astral structure. Then the flakes gradually disappeared, and Saturn returned through the same stages into the darkness of pralaya.[14]

Saturn reappeared as Sun, and with it came the human being, the ancient inhabitant of the universe. In the meantime, the human being had gained the power to separate something from out of himself. Finer substances he retained within himself so that he might evolve to a higher level. In this way he formed the minerals from out of himself, but these minerals were living minerals. On the Sun, the human being evolved in such a way that the etheric body could be added. There were thus two kingdoms on the Sun, the mineral kingdom and the plant kingdom. But these plant forms were quite different from those we know today.

The Sun was a body of light, composed of light-ether; the human being was plantlike, his head directed towards the centre of the Sun. When the Sun had evolved to its limit, it disappeared into the darkness of pralaya and eventually reappeared as Moon.[15]

The Old Moon had no solid mineral kingdom. It was a globe which, instead of a solid earth crust, had something like a living and inwardly growing peaty mass. This living foundation was permeated with woody structures out of which grew the plant kingdom, as it then was. These plants, however, were really a sort of 'plant-animal'; they were able to feel and under pressure would have experienced pain. And the human being in the animal kingdom of the time was not like any animal of today; he was half-way between animal and the human being. He was of a higher order than our present animals and could carry out his impulses in a much more systematic way.

On Saturn, the physical body of the human being was a body of warmth; on the Sun, the gaseous condition condensed to 'air'. Now, in Moon evolution, when the astral was poured in, the moment was reached when the physical attained a further stage of condensation. The human physical body thus came to assume a form composed of three organic structures, distinct from one another in their substance. The densest was a 'water body'; this was permeated by airy currents, and warmth effects also continued to pervade the whole. After disappearing into pralaya, the Moon reappeared as the earth.

In Genesis,[16] we find a theory of evolution compared with which the proud doctrines of today are mere fantasy. For Genesis guides us to the inwardness of creation, shows us what has to take place at the supersensory level before the human being can advance to sensory existence.

Thus while the other beings had already condensed physically in air and water, the human being had still to remain in etheric existence, and it was his condensation to the stage of the etheric body that took place in the period alluded to as the fifth day of creation. On the fifth day we still do not find the human being among the physical earth beings. It is not until the sixth day that we find the human being actually among the earth beings.

If you enter a space and find there differentiated currents of warmth not as dense as gas, that must still be described as physical existence. The human being on the sixth day was not to be found in solid, fleshly form. He was to be found in physical form, as an earth being, but only in the first manifestation of the physical, as a human being of warmth.[17]

At the beginning of the development of the earth there was a state of soul and spirit; then came an astral state, then an etheric state, and then came the physical states, first warmth and then air. Even as regards the point of time when, after the six 'days' of creation, we are told 'And the Lord God ... breathed into his nostrils the breath of life' we have not understood our own origin so long as we believe that a human being of flesh and blood was already there — unless we think of the human being at that moment as consisting only of warmth and air. The coarser is derived from the finer, not the finer from the coarser. When we have grasped this, we shall understand why it is that in so many accounts of creation the incarnation of the human being is represented as a descent from the periphery of the earth. When the Bible itself, after the 'days' of creation, speaks of Paradise, we must look for the deeper meaning behind this, and only spiritual science will enable us to understand the truth.

The emergence of modern consciousness

Our Atlantean ancestors differed more from present-day human beings than someone would imagine whose knowledge is confined wholly to the world of the senses.[18] This difference extended not only to external appearance but also to spiritual faculties. Their knowledge, their technical skills, indeed their entire civilization differed from what can be observed today. If we go back to the first periods of Atlantean humanity, we find a mental capacity quite different from ours. Logical reason, the power of arithmetical combining were totally absent. On the other hand, they had a highly developed memory.

In the Atlantean time, the human being was not unconscious at night but could perceive just as he perceived by day. By day he perceived the first traces of what we today see as the world of sense perceptions. By night he was the companion of the divine spiritual beings. He needed no proof of the existence of gods, just as we today need no proof of the existence of minerals. The gods were his companions; he himself was a spiritual being during the night. In his astral body and ego he wandered about the spiritual world.

The Atlantean did not raise himself to his God through concepts and ideas. He discerned something holy in nature as a keynote of the divine. If he wished to express what he heard this way, he would embody it in a sound similar to the Chinese T-A-O. For the Atlantean this was the sound which pervaded the whole of nature. When he touched a leaf, or saw a flash of lightning, he was aware that part of the Godhead was displayed before him. Just as we make contact with some element in a human being's soul when we shake hands with him, so the Atlantean, when he took hold of a form in nature, felt that he was touching the body of the Godhead.

But then the type of thinking associated with logic and mathematical calculation began to develop, and the more it did so, the more clairvoyance faded away. People began to concern themselves more with what the senses could perceive, so nature was increasingly divested of divinity. In proportion as they achieved the gift of exact sense-observation, they ceased to understand nature as the body of the Godhead. Gradually they came to see only the body of the world and not its soul. But as the result of this, a yearning for the divine arose once more in the human being. He came to realize that he must seek for God with his spirit. That is in fact the meaning of the word 'religion': to try to re-establish a connection with the Godhead; *religere* means to reunite.

Now there are various ways of finding the Godhead. The Indians, who were the first sub-race of the Aryan race,[19] took the following way. Certain God-inspired messengers of Manu, called the Holy Rishis, became the teachers of ancient Indian culture. No poetry or tradition tells us about this—it is known only through what has been handed down orally in the occult schools. Poems such as the Vedas and the *Bhagavadgita*, wonderful as they are, are of much later origin. The ancient Indian felt in his heart that external nature as he saw it was unreal, and that behind it the Godhead was concealed. The name he gave to this Godhead was Brahman, the hidden God. The whole external world was thus for him an illusion,

deception, maya. Whereas the Atlantean could still discern the Godhead in every leaf, the Indian said: 'The
Godhead is no longer apparent in the outer world. I must
descend into my inner being and seek for him in my heart;
I must follow after him towards a higher spiritual
condition.'

The second sub-race, that of the ancient Persians, had a
different mission, although its culture had its origins in
the clear purpose of Manu. Long before the time of Zarathustra, Persia had an ancient culture of which only an
oral tradition survives. The idea began to take a hold
among people that external reality was an image of the
divine which must not be turned away from but shaped
anew. The Persian wished to transform nature by work; he
became a farmer. He moved out of the quiet realm of
world-renouncing thoughts and learnt from the resistance
he encountered that the outer world was not wholly maya.
Alongside with the world of the spirit he found a real
world in which work had to be done.[20]

If we wish to characterize the difference between the
Indian and Persian cultures, we may say that a member of
the Persian culture felt the physical to be not merely a
burden but a task to be fulfilled. He also looked up into the
regions of light, into the spiritual worlds, but he turned his
gaze back into the physical world and in his soul he saw
how everything divides into the powers of light and the
powers of darkness. The physical world became for him a
field of work. The Persian said to himself, 'There is the
beneficent fullness of light, the god Ahura Mazda or

Ormuzd, and there are the dark powers under the leadership of Angramainyush or Ahriman.

The conquest of the physical plane proceeded further in the third cultural epoch, in the Egyptian-Babylonian-Assyrian-Chaldean culture. At this time, hardly anything remained of the ancient repugnance with which the physical world was felt to be maya. The Chaldeans looked up to the heavens, and the light of the stars was not merely maya for them; it was the script that the gods had imprinted on the physical plane. On the paths of the stars the Chaldean priest pursued his way back into the spiritual worlds, and when he was initiated, when he learned to know all the beings who inhabited the planets and the stars, he lifted up his eyes and said, 'What I see with my eyes when I gaze up to the heavens is the outer expression of what is given me by occult vision, by initiation.'

The fourth epoch, the Graeco-Latin, is the period when the human being came even more into contact with the physical plane. In this time the human being progressed so far that he not only saw the script of the gods in the physical world, but he also inserted his own self, his spiritual individuality, into the objective world. Such artistic creations as we find in Greece were not known earlier. That the human being could portray himself in sculpture, creating something like his physical self — this was achieved in the fourth cultural period.[21]

In the Atlantean time, the human being lost almost entirely the feeling of being at home with the gods, and when the great catastrophe was past, a great part of humankind had completely lost the natural ability to gaze into the spiritual world at night. But in place of this they gained the capacity of seeing ever more sharply by day, so that the objects around them appeared in ever clearer outlines. Among the human beings who had remained behind, the gift of clairvoyance was still preserved, even into the post-Atlantean cultures. At the time when Christianity was founded, remnants of this clairvoyance still existed, and even today there are occasional persons who have preserved it as a natural gift.

When the human being of today conceives a thought, he ascribes it to his own activity of thinking. He forms chains of thoughts in accordance with rules of logic. The human being of ancient times received these thoughts. He paid no heed at all to how the connections between thoughts should be formulated, for they came to him as revelations. But this meant that he did not live in his thoughts in the way we live in ours. We regard our thoughts as the possession of our soul; we know that we have worked to acquire them.

The human being said to himself as he contemplated his thoughts: 'A divine being from a higher world has descended into me. I partake of the thoughts which in reality other beings are thinking — beings who are higher than the human being but who inspire me, who live in me, who give me these thoughts. I can therefore only regard the thoughts as having been vouchsafed to me by grace from above.' It was because the human being of old held this view that he felt the need at certain seasons to make an offering of these thoughts to higher beings.

The knowledge contained in paganism had its source in the ancient mysteries and, although according to modern scholarship it bears a mythical, pictorial character, it must be emphasized that all the imagery, all the pictures that have come down to posterity from this ancient paganism are the fruits of profound insight.

Recalling the many treasures of this supersensible lore, it will be obvious that here we are dealing with a primeval wisdom, a wisdom underlying all the thinking, all the perceptions and feelings of ancient peoples. A kind of echo of this primeval wisdom, a tradition in which it was enshrined, survived here and there in secret societies — actually in a healthy form until the end of the eighteenth century and the beginning of the nineteenth.

Now this ancient wisdom has one particular characteristic of which sight must never be lost. It has one characteristic on account of which Judaism, the smaller stream then making preparation for Christianity, had to be introduced.

If this ancient paganism is rightly understood, it will be found to contain sublime, deeply penetrating wisdom, but no moral impulses for human action. These impulses were not really essential to the human being, for unlike what now passes as human knowledge, human insight, this old pagan wisdom gave him the feeling of being integrated into the whole cosmos. A human being moving about the earth not only felt himself composed of the substances and forces present around him in earthly life, in the mineral, plant and animal kingdoms, but he felt that the forces operating, for example, in the movements of the stars and the sun, were playing into him. This feeling of being a member of the whole cosmos was not a mere abstraction, for from the mysteries he received instructions based on the laws of the stars for his actions and whole conduct of life. This ancient star-wisdom was in no way akin to the arithmetical astrology sometimes considered valuable today, but it was a wisdom voiced by the initiates in such a way that impulses for individual action and conduct went forth from the mysteries. Not only did the human being feel safe and secure within the all-prevailing wisdom of the cosmos, but those whom he recognized as the initiates of the mysteries imparted this wisdom in instructions for his actions from morning till evening on given days of the year. Yet neither Chaldean nor Egyptian wisdom contained a single moral impulse from what had been imparted by the initiates in this way. The moral impulse in its real sense was prepared by Judaism and then further developed in Christianity.

The significance of changes in nutrition

Human beings in earlier times could absorb food substance in the same way that today the lungs take in air. At that time threads of suction connected the human being with the whole of nature around him, somewhat in the manner in which today the embryo is nourished in the body of the mother. This was the old form of nourishment on the earth. A relic of this is the suckling of mammals, and milk is like the nourishment humankind took in pre-Lemurian times. It is the old food of the gods, the first form of nourishment on the earth. At that time the nature of the earth was such that everywhere this nourishment could be sucked from it. Thus milk is a product of the first form of human food. When the physical constitution of the human being was nearer to the divine, he sucked milk out of his surroundings.

Before the time when milk was imbibed from nature, there was an age in which the earth was still united with the sun. Everything irradiated with sunlight — blossoms and fruits of the plants — belongs to the sun. Formerly they planted themselves into the sun with their blossoms. When the earth separated from the sun they retained their old character: they again turned their blossoms towards the sun. The human being is the plant in reverse. That part of the plant which grows above the earth has the same relationship to the sun as milk has to the moon. Alongside milk nourishment there arose a kind of plant nourishment, namely, from the upper parts of the plant. This was the second form of human food.

Thus when the Lemurian age was approaching its end, two human types faced each other: the one kind, the sons of the moon, bred animals and nourished themselves from what the animals produced, from their milk; the second kind fed on plants, on the produce of the earth. This fact is portrayed in the story of Cain and Abel. Abel is a shepherd, Cain a tiller of the soil: Abel represented the moon race and Cain the sun race.

When we go back into the most ancient times we find no nourishment at all except milk, the food which the human being received from living animals. Now we come from the Lemurian to the Atlantean age. With the Atlanteans, something new appeared. They began to eat food that was not taken from what was living, but from what was dead. They consumed what had yielded up life. This is a very important transition in human evolution. Through the fact that human beings nourished themselves from the lifeless it became possible to make the transition to egohood. The human being became independent through eating what is dead. He took the lifeless into himself in various forms. The first to do so were the developing hunting peoples who killed animals. Later, peoples arose who ate not only what was ripened by the sun but what ripened below the surface of the earth. This is just as lifeless as the dead animal. The moon force itself is still in milk, which is connected with the life process, whereas the human being absorbs the forces of what is dying when he eats what is dead. Equally dead is that part of the plant that grows below the surface of the earth, that is not illuminated and warmed through by the life principle of the sun.

Another form of food was added which did not exist earlier. The human being introduced into his food what was purely mineral, what he took out of the earth, salt and so on. In his food, therefore, he passed through the three kingdoms. This is approximately the course which Atlantean civilization passed through in regard to nourishment. Firstly came the hunting peoples, then the farming peoples and thirdly the development of mining, which brought to light what is under the earth. Everything of the nature of salt is the dead nature of the mineral kingdom that remains over from the past.

Now we come to the fifth human race.[22] In the fifth root race the most outstanding addition is what was gained from minerals by means of a chemical process. This is indicated in Genesis. Chemistry was applied to plants, to fruit, leading to the creation of wine. Therefore the Bible tells us that Noah, the original ancestor of the post-Diluvian race, became intoxicated by wine.

Wine had first made its appearance with the Persians. Here, however, wine was still something quite secular. Only gradually did it find its way into ritual, into the Dionysus cult. Wine cuts human beings off from everything spiritual.[23] Whoever takes wine cannot attain the spiritual. He can know nothing of Atma, Buddhi and Manas, of what is lasting, of what reincarnates. This had to be. The whole course of human evolution is a descent and a reascent. And it was in order that he should come right down onto the physical plane that the Dionysian cult made its appearance. The human body had to be prepared for materialism through the Dionysian cult; this was why a religion had to appear that changed water into wine. Formerly wine was strictly forbidden to the priests; they could experience Atma, Buddhi and Manas. Now a religion had to arise that led right down onto the physical plane.

Meat is taken from that kingdom which is specifically

earthly, it is not taken from the actual life process of the human or animal being like milk. Meat really fetters the human being to the earth. It makes him into a creature of the earth, so that to the extent that he permeates his organism with the effects of meat he deprives himself of the forces which would enable him to free himself from the earth. Through a meat diet he binds himself strongly to the earth. Whilst milk enables him to belong to the earth as a transitory stage in his development, meat condemns him — unless he is raised up by something else.

What part of the potato do we eat? The part that is below, the tuber; and tubers, roots and so on are those parts of the plant which are least digested in the intestines. Fruits are digested in the intestines. Now we eat a potato and it goes into the stomach and the intestines. It cannot be digested there but goes up with the blood undigested. So when it arrives at the appropriate layer of the brain, it is not in the fine condition of rye or wheat which can straight away be sent into the rest of the body; it has to be processed and digested there in the brain. So if we eat rye or wheat bread which we digest thoroughly in our stomach and intestines, we do not have to burden our head with digesting it. It can be distributed throughout the body straight away. If we eat potatoes, the head has to serve as a digestive organ. So if the human being eats too many potatoes — which has happened to an increasing extent since the potato was introduced into Europe and became important — the head becomes less capable of thinking and the human being loses the capacity to think with the middle of the brain; he thinks only with the frontal part. This frontal part, which depends on salts, causes us to become more and more materialistically intellectual. Real spiritual thoughts cannot be thought by the frontal part of the brain. It is a fact that inner thinking in Europe regressed from the moment that the potato took hold.

2. Cosmos as the Source of Life

Knowledge of astronomy is nowadays presented as if it were an extension of geography or physics instead of having a profound connection with our existence. The heavenly bodies are well named, for Steiner makes clear that they are the homes or visible garments of groups of spirit beings whose creative energies have been spent on the furtherance of the human race throughout successive epochs. As the human being has slowly evolved, so have these beings – the attainment of the tasks has enabled them to rise higher. They can be grouped hierarchically and might be considered as serving the almighty Creator Being or Godhead like parts of an immense organism.

A certain belt of stars traversed by sun and moon forms the zodiac. This has a special connection with life on the earth. While human beings are largely emancipated from such influences, animals and plants are more directly affected, and when sun or moon passes in front of a zodiacal constellation its cosmic influence is to some degree blocked – as with an eclipse. There is therefore a constant need for living creatures to be compensating for deficiencies in outer forces, which calls forth a certain effort.

Steiner's view of the sun is of special interest. We are encouraged to think of the sun as a suctional force drawing in etheric substance from the different parts of the universe, with solar activity being the result. The sun also causes the planets to follow it in the course of time rather than simply circulate around it. We finally look in more detail at the formative elements of life – earth, water, air and warmth – emanating as ethers from the different constellations as the Greeks and Asian people earlier recognized. We need to understand the true meanings which these words had for ancient people and we need to appreciate the deeds of spiritual beings in bringing about what we call 'substance'.

Stars and the significance of the zodiac

If we look up to the stars, we can say that something streams from them that can be perceived by the human being's sense organs here on earth. But what we behold when we gaze at the stars is not of the same nature as what we perceive on the earth in the mineral, plant and animal kingdoms. In reality it proceeds from beings of intelligence and will whose life is bound up with those stars. The effects appear to be physical because the stars are at a distance. They are not in reality physical at all. What you actually see are the activities of beings of will and intelligence in the stars. I have spoken to you of the ingenious description of the sun given by astrophysicists. But if it were possible to journey to the sun it would be found with amazement that nothing of what is to be expected from these physical descriptions exists. The descriptions are merely a composite picture of solar phenomena. What we see is in reality the working of will and intelligence which at a distance appears as light.

Let us try for a moment to consider space alone, and out of the whole visible heavens let us consider the regions that comprise the zodiac. Let us consider the directions to which we look in the heavens when we turn, for instance, towards Aries (Ram) in the zodiac; then Taurus, Gemini, Cancer, Leo, Virgo, Libra, Scorpio, Sagittarius, Capricorn, Aquarius and Pisces. All we have to note, in the first place, is that the space that lies before us as our visible universe is divided in this way. The signs merely denote the boundary of a certain section of space.

Now we must not imagine that these directions of space can be treated in such a manner that one might say: 'There is empty space, and I just draw a line somewhere into it.' Such a thing as mathematics calls 'space' simply does not exist; but everywhere are lines of force, directions of force, and these are not equal, they vary, they are differentiated. We can distinguish between these twelve regions by realizing that if we turn in the direction of the sign of Aries, the force we experience is a different one than it would be had we faced the sign of Libra or Cancer. In each direction the force differs. The human being will not admit this as long as he lives merely in the world of the senses; but as soon as he ascends to the imaginative life of the soul, he no longer experiences the directions in space as the same when facing Aries or Cancer, but feels their influence upon him as greatly differentiated.[24]

People are unaware what a specialized thing the sun is. The sun is not really the same when in the course of a year or a day it shines onto the earth from Taurus, or from

Cancer, or the other constellations. In each case it is different. It is comparative nonsense to speak of the sun in general terms—albeit, pardonable nonsense. We should really speak of Aries-sun, Taurus-sun, Cancer-sun, Leo-sun, and so on. For the sun is a different being in each case. Moreover, the resultant influence depends both on the daily course and on the yearly course of the sun, as determined by its position in the vernal point.

The sun maintains its power through the fact that it comes into connection with the different regions of the universe. It also means something different for the earth if the sun's light is strengthened or weakened by the other planets of our planetary system. And here different relationships arise in regard to the different planets; the relationships to the 'outer planets'—Mars, Jupiter and Saturn—are different from those to the 'inner planets'—Mercury, Venus and moon.

It is clear that our metabolic forces still retain a certain connection with the rhythm of our daily life. The forces of form have solidified. Now consider the animal instead of the human being. Here we shall find a much more complete dependence upon the macrocosm. The human being has grown out of or beyond this dependence. Ancient wisdom therefore referred to the zodiac or 'animal circle', not to the 'human being circle', as corresponding to formative forces. These forces manifest themselves in the animal kingdom in a great variety of forms, while in the human being they manifest essentially in one form encompassing the whole human race; but they are the forces of the animal kingdom, and as we evolve beyond them and become the human being, we must go out beyond the zodiac. Beyond the zodiac lies that upon which we, as human beings, are dependent in a higher sense than we are upon all that exists within the zodiac, that is, within the circle of the fixed stars. Beyond the zodiac is that which corresponds to our ego.

With the astral body — which the animal also possesses — we are fettered to a dependence upon the macrocosm, and the building up of the astral vehicle takes place in accordance with the will of the stars. But with our 'I' or ego we transcend the zodiac.

Here we have the principle upon which we have gained our freedom. Within the zodiac we cannot sin, any more than can the animals; we begin to sin as soon as we carry our actions beyond the zodiac. This happens when we do things that make us free from our connection with universal formative forces, when we enter into a relationship with regions exterior to the zodiac or the region of fixed stars. And this is the essential content of the human ego.

You see, we may measure the universe in so far as it appears to us a visible and temporal thing, we may measure its full extent through space to the outermost fixed stars, and all that takes place by way of movement in time in this starry heaven, and we may consider all this in its relation to the human being; but in the human being something is being fulfilled that occurs outside this space and outside this time, outside all that takes place in the astral. Beyond the latter there is no 'natural necessity', but only what is intimately connected with our moral nature and moral actions. Within the zodiac we are unable to evolve our moral nature; but in so far as we evolve it, we record it into the macrocosm beyond the zodiac. All that we do remains and works in the world.

Now the stars we see may be further away from or closer to the moon. Looking at the stars we see the moon pass through the starry heavens. But whilst some constellations are positioned in such a way that the moon always passes through them, it does not pass through others. So if you consider Hercules, for instance, the moon does not pass through it. But if you look at the Lion, then the moon always passes through the Lion at given intervals. Twelve constellations have the special characteristic that they form the path taken by the moon and also by the sun. We may say, therefore, that the twelve constellations Ram, Bull, Twins, Crab, Lion, Virgin, Scales, Scorpion, Archer, Goat, Water Carrier and Fishes mark the path of the moon. It always passes through them and not through the other constellations. We are thus always able to say that at any particular time the moon, if it is in the sky, is in one constellation or another, but only a constellation that is part of the zodiac.

Now I want you to consider that everything there is by way of stars in the sky has a definite influence on the earth as a whole and specifically also on the human being. The human being truly depends not only on what exists here on earth but also on the stars that are there in the heavens.

Think of some star or constellation up there. It rises in

the evening and sets in the morning. It is there all the time, and always influences the human being. But think of another constellation, the Twins, let us say, or the Lion. The moon passes that way. The moment it passes that way it covers up the Twins or the Lion. I see only the moon and not the Twins. At that moment they cannot influence the earth, because their influence is blocked. And so we have stars everywhere in the sky that are never blocked out, either by the sun or by the moon, and always have an influence on the earth. And we have stars which the moon passes, and the sun also passes them. These are covered up from time to time and their influence then stops. We are therefore able to say that the Lion is a constellation in the zodiac and has a particular influence on the human being. It does not have this influence if the moon is in front of it. At that time the human being is free of the Lion's influence, the Lion's influence does not affect him.

Now just imagine you are terribly lazy and will not walk unless someone gives you a push from behind, and you have to walk. He drives you on, and that is his influence. But imagine I do not permit him to influence you; he cannot give you a push. Then you are not subject to the influence; and if you want to walk you have to do it yourself.

Human beings need these influences. The Lion constellation has a particular influence on the human being. It has this influence for as long as it is not covered up by the moon or the sun. But let us take this further. Again consider an analogy from life. Let us say you want

to know something. When you are little you do not want
to think for yourself, you ask your tutor. But if the tutor
has gone out, so that you do not have your tutor available
at the moment and have to do your homework, then you
have to find the power in yourself. You have to recall
things for yourself.

The Lion continually influences human beings except
when it is covered by the moon. Then the influence is not
there. When the moon blocks the Lion's influence, the
human being must develop using his own resources.[25]
Someone able to develop his own strong Lion influence
when the moon covers the constellation may thus be
called a Lion person. Someone able to develop particularly
the influence in the constellation of the Crab when this is
covered up is a Crab person. People develop the one or the
other more strongly depending on their inner constitution.

You see, thus, that the constellations of the zodiac are
special, for sometimes their influence exists and sometimes it does not. The passage of the moon through the
constellations at four-week intervals means that there is
always a time in a four-week period when some
constellation of the zodiac does not have an influence.
With other constellations the influence is always the same.
In earlier times people took these influences that came
from the heavens very seriously.[26] The zodiac was therefore more important to them than other constellations. The
others have a continuous influence which does not
change. But with the zodiac we may say that the influence
changes depending on whether one of its constellations is

covered over or not. Because of this, the influence of the zodiac on the earth has always been the subject of special study. And so you see why the zodiac is more important when we study the starry heavens than are other stars.

The sun and its planetary relationships

The sun is not a ball of gas; but in that place where the sun is there is something less than empty space — a sucking, absorbing body, in fact, while all around it is that which exerts pressure. Consequently what comes to us from the sun is nothing to do with any product of combustion in the sun, but is a reflection, a raying back of all that the universe has radiated to it.

The location of the sun is emptier than empty space. This can be said of all parts of the universe where we find ether. For this reason it is so difficult for physicists to speak of ether, for they think that ether is also matter, though more rarefied than ordinary matter.

Anyone who believes that in ether we are dealing merely with a 'rarefying' process is like someone who says: 'I have here a purse full of money; I repeatedly take from it and the money becomes less and less. I take away still more till at last none remains, nothing is left.' But in fact one can continue! The 'nothing' can become less still; for if we get into debt, our money becomes less than nothing. In the same way not only does matter become empty space, but it becomes negative, less than nothing, emptier than emptiness; it assumes a 'sucking' nature. Ether is sucking, absorbing. Matter presses, ether absorbs. The sun is an absorbing, sucking sphere, and wherever ether is present we have this force of suction.

It is simply not possible to apply to conditions on the sun or to cosmic space notions that have been derived from heat phenomena observable in the terrestrial sphere. It will be understood that the sun's corona and similar phenomena have antecedents not included in the observations made under terrestrial conditions. Just as our thinking leads us astray when we abandon observation and theorize our way through a world of atoms and molecules, so we fall into error when we go out into the macrocosm and apply to the sun what we have determined from observations under earthly conditions. Such a method has led to the belief that the sun is a kind of glowing ball of gas, but the sun is by no means a glowing ball of gas.

Whilst on the surface of the earth an eruption or the like will naturally be interpreted as tending up and outwards, a process on the sun—a sunspot for example—must be interpreted rather as tending from the outside in. Continuing this line of thought, just as we have to imagine that if we went through and beneath the surface of the earth we should get into dense matter, so we have to imagine that if we moved from outside the sun towards the sun's interior we should come into an ever more rarified state of matter. Look at the earth and the whole way it is placed into the universe. It manifests as so much conceivable matter in the universe. Not so the sun. Here we can only come near the truth if we imagine that as we go from the circumference towards the interior we get ever more remote from conceivable matter and ever more and more into the inconceivable. We have precisely the opposite behaviour from the earth as we draw near its centre.[27] The sun must be conceived of as a hollowing out of cosmic matter, a hollow space, a hollow sphere enveloped by matter, in contrast to the earth where we have denser matter enveloped by more rarefied. As to the earth, we think of air around it. Air is outside and denser matter inside. For the sun it is the opposite; as we go inwards we go from relatively denser matter into more rarefied and at long last into the very negation of matter. Anyone who approaches the phenomena with an open mind and puts them all together will recognize that this is so. The sun is not only a more rarefied heavenly body of material characteristics less dense than earthly matter, but if we call the earth's material characteristics positive, then in the sun — in the sun's interior — we have negative matter.

As compared with positive matter, negative matter is suctional. And if you now conceive of the sun as a suctional force, you need no further explanation of gravitation. The movement of earth and sun is such that the earth follows the sun in the same path, in the same direction. Here, then, you have the cosmic relation between sun and earth. The sun as a gathering of suctional forces moves ahead and the earth is drawn after it by this suctional force, moving through cosmic space in the same course and in the same direction in which the sun is propelled forward.

It is not enough to adopt the methods of the Copernican system and simply draw ellipses intended to show the paths of Saturn, Jupiter, Mars, earth, Venus, Mercury and sun. What is needed, on the contrary, is to look at the laws that are active in the worlds that are physically perceptible and see how these laws are interwoven by an altogether different set of laws, and that especially the present moon in its motion presents something that is in no way causally connected with the rest of the stellar system, as would be the case if the moon were a part of that system in the same way as other planets. The moon, however, is related to quite another world which interpenetrates ours and which represents the breathing process of our universe as the sun represents the interpenetration of our universe by the ether.

It is Newtonian science that has driven us so far into materialism because it seizes on the uttermost abstractions. It speaks of a force of gravitation. The sun, it says, attracts the earth, or the earth attracts the moon; a force of attraction exists between these bodies, like some invisible cable. But if really nothing but this force of attraction existed, there would be no cause for the moon to revolve round the earth or the earth round the sun; the moon would simply fall onto the earth. This would indeed have happened ages ago if gravitation alone were acting; or the earth would have fallen into the sun. It is therefore quite impossible for us to look to gravitation alone for the means of explaining the imagined or actual motions of celestial bodies.

Modern astronomy endeavours with all manner of arguments to speak of an elliptic path of the earth around the sun. It asserts that this motion was first initiated by that tangential propulsion of which I spoke yesterday in connection with the sun's gravitational attraction. But astronomy cannot, and does not, deny the fact that when speaking of attraction not only does the sun attract the earth, but the earth must also attract the sun. This, however, obliges us to conclude that we cannot speak of an elliptical orbit of the earth around the sun, for if the attraction be mutual we cannot have a one-sided motion of the earth around the sun, but both of them must revolve round a neutral point. In other words, this orbit cannot take place in a manner that would allow us to look on the sun's centre as the pivot, but the pivot must be a neutral point situated between the centre of the sun and the centre of the earth. In telling you this, I am not raising objections to astronomy, I am merely telling you what you can find for yourselves in astronomical books. Thus we are compelled to admit the existence—somehow or other—of a pivot between the two spheres.

Elementary conditions and spiritual beings

Anyone who wishes to get to the bottom of things has to ask himself which of the hierarchies caused the more rarefied warmth-substance to turn into denser air. It is the same Spirits of Will who sacrificed the warmth substance out of themselves who brought this about. We may describe their activity by saying that during Saturn evolution they were so advanced as to be able to allow their own substance to flow out as warmth, so advanced as to be able to offer their own substance as a sacrifice, so advanced that their fire streamed into the planetary existence of Saturn. Then during Sun evolution they condensed their fire into the gaseous element. But it was also they who during Moon evolution condensed their gaseous element to water. During Earth evolution they further condensed their watery element into the earth element, into a solid. Thus, when we look upon the solid matter in the world, we have to say to ourselves that in this solid matter forces are at work which alone make its existence possible, forces whose very being flowed out from Saturn as warmth and whose effluence has become denser and denser until it has now reached the solid state, held together by their power.

You must get used to the thought that in what lies nearest to us, and which we often regard as very lowly, we sometimes meet very high and exalted beings. It is easy to say of the solid element that it is only matter. Perhaps some may be tempted to say that it is no concern of the spiritual investigator — that matter is a low level of existence. Why should we bother with it? We pass beyond and above matter into the spiritual. Anyone who thinks in this way forgets that through countless ages high, exalted

spiritual beings have worked in the object of his contempt
to bring it into this solid state. Actually, when we penetrate through external matter, through the elementary
covering of the earth, to what has made this earth covering
solid, it would be natural to feel the deepest reverence for
the exalted beings we call the Spirits of Will, who have
laboured so long in this earth element to build up the solid
ground upon which we tread, and which we ourselves
bear within us in the earthly constituents of our physical
bodies. It is these Spirits of Will, whom in Christian esotericism we also call the Thrones, who have in fact con-
structed—or rather condensed—the solid ground upon
which we walk.

If we now reascend from the solid to the watery condition, we may reflect that it took longer to build up and
densify the earth element than the watery. Hence we have
to look for the fundamental forces of the watery element in
beings of a lower hierarchy. For the condensation of the
watery element, as it is at work around us in the
elementary state, needed only the activity of the Spirits of
Wisdom, the Kyriotetes, the Dominions.

When we ascend to the airy element, we see a still lower
hierarchy at work. In the airy formations around us, to the
extent that they are caused by forces underlying them, we
also see the effect of the activity of certain spirits of the
hierarchies. Just as the Spirits of Wisdom work in the
water, so the Spirits of Movement—the Dynamis—are at
work in the airy forms. And when we come to warmth, to
the next stage of rarefaction, then it is the next lower

hierarchy, the Spirits of Form — the Exusiai — who live and weave within it, the same spirits whom we refer to as the Elohim. Up to now we have, from quite a different direction, characterized the Spirits of Form as the spirits who brooded in the warmth element. When we trace the order of the hierarchies in the downward direction from the Spirits of Will, through the Spirits of Wisdom and the Spirits of Movement, we come back to our Elohim, the Spirits of Form. You see how everything fits together, if the threads are woven in the right way. If you now try to bring sensitive and perceptive feeling into all this, you will say that behind all we see around us through our senses there lies an elementary existence: an earth element, but within this element there live the Spirits of Will; a fluid element, in which live the Spirits of Wisdom; an airy element, in which live the Spirits of Movement; and a warmth element, in which live the Spirits of Form, the Elohim.

The nature of the four primal elements

It is totally wrong to think that we can carry our own meaning of the words earth, water and air over into ancient writings in which Greek influence was dominant and assume that the corresponding words have the same meaning there. When we come across the word 'water' in ancient writings, we must translate it with our word 'fluidity', and the word 'earth' with our word 'solids'.

Only in this way can we correctly translate the ancient writings. But a profound significance is implicit in this. The use of the word earth to indicate solids implies especially that this solid condition falls under the laws prevailing on the planet earth. Solids were designated as earth because it was desired to convey this idea: when a body is solid it is under the influence of earthly laws in every respect. On the other hand, when a body was spoken of as water, then it was not merely under earthly laws but influenced by the entire planetary system.

It was therefore felt that only solid bodies, designated as earth, were solely under the earth's system of laws, and that when a body melted it was influenced from outside the earth. And when a gaseous body was called air, the feeling was that such a body was under the unifying influence of the sun.

Earthly air beings were looked upon in this way: the forces of the sun were essentially active in their configuration, their inner arrangement and substance. Ancient physics had a cosmic character. It was willing to take into account the forces actually present.

The consciousness of certain things was completely lost in the period extending from the fifteenth to the seventeenth centuries — the consciousness that our earth is a member of the solar system as a whole, and that consequently every single thing on the earth is connected with the solar system as a whole.[28]

When we proceed from solid bodies to water, we are obliged to extend our considerations not only to what actually lies before us; in order to get an intelligent idea of the nature of water, we must extend such considerations to include the water of the whole earth and to think of this as a unity in relation to the central point of the earth. To observe a 'fragment' of water as a physical entity is as absurd as to consider a cut-off fragment of my little finger as an organism. The fragment would die at once. It only has meaning as an organism if it is considered in its relation to the whole organism. Water does not in itself have the meaning that the solid has in itself. It has meaning only in relation to the whole earth. And so it is with all liquids on the earth.

And again, when we pass on from the fluid to the gaseous, we come to understand that the gaseous removes itself from the earthly domain. It does not form normal surfaces. It is part of everything that is not terrestrial. In other words, we must not merely look on the earth for what is active in a gas; we must consider what surrounds the earth, we must go out into space and seek there the forces involved. When we wish to learn the laws of the gaseous state, we become involved in nothing less than astronomical considerations.

Thus you see how these things are related to the whole terrestrial scheme when we examine the phenomena that up to now we have simply gathered together. And when we come to a point such as the melting or boiling point, very significant things arise. For when we consider the melting point, we pass from the terrestrial condition of a solid body, in which it determines its own form and relations, to something that includes the whole earth. The earth begins to take the solid captive when the solid passes into the fluid state. From its own kingdom, the solid enters the terrestrial kingdom as a whole when we reach melting point. It ceases to have individuality. And when we carry the fluid over into the gaseous state, then we come to the point where the connection with the earth as shown by the formation of a liquid surface is loosened. The instant we go from a liquid to a gas, the body loosens itself from the earthly domain and enters the realm of the extra-terrestrial.[29] We must consider the forces active in a gas as having escaped from the earth. When we study these phenomena, therefore, we cannot avoid passing from the ordinary physical and terrestrial sphere into the cosmic. For we are no longer in contact with reality if our attention is not turned to what is actually working in the things themselves.

We can say that in solids we discover the images of the fluid state, in fluid we discover the images of the gaseous state, in the gaseous state we discover images of warmth.

When we have followed further this path of thinking, we will have made an important step. We will have advanced to the point where we have a picture in the gaseous state, which is accessible to human observation, of heat manifestations and even of the real nature of heat itself. We then gain the possibility, if we are seeking the images of heat in the gaseous state correctly, to explain the nature of heat even though we are obliged to admit that it is an unknown entity to us.

If we consider correctly the things that are revealed to us by bodies under the influence of heat and pressure, we will see how we arrive at what the gases can reveal to us — the real nature of heat. In cooling, the being of heat penetrates further into the liquid and solid states. We have to pursue the nature of this heat entity also in these states, although we can do it best in the gaseous condition where it is more evident.

3. Plants and the Living Earth

The life of plants is fundamental to the life of the earth, as plants are for the earth organism what senses are for the human being. The opposing direction of root and leaf development expresses the vertical orientation between the earth's centre and the sun, between the soul and spiritual aspects of plants. When we look at mineral matter, now crystalline, we should develop the feeling that this has once been alive and plantlike. In the amazing patterns of ice crystals we see revealed the same formative processes which work through all physical substance, whether mineral or organic.

The earth, as with all living organisms, experiences a breathing process connected with the diurnal and annual cycle of the sun. During summer we tend to think that nature is most awake whereas the soul of living things is more asleep at this time. It is in summer, when the soul of the earth and all its creatures is drawn out into the cosmos that the light beings of the sun experience a consciousness of the earth. Steiner tells us that the crystallizing forces drawn into the earth in winter – and at night-time – together with the warmth and light forces in the soil from the previous summer, all affect the new season's growth.

As plants do not have a self-contained astral body, astrality – as Steiner refers to it – is concentrated outside them. This astrality is part of the earth's astral body but is modified according to the nature of each species. It is particularly intense

*in the airy environment of trees, which as a result have a bene-
ficial effect on a wide area around them. Contrary to the conventional wisdom on fertilization and seed formation, Steiner
tells us that seeds can only be formed as a result of a cosmic image
of the plant being taken up by a sap layer known as the cambium.
He explains that while all plants have tree-forming tendencies,
the cambium of a tree is the equivalent of the root system of an
annual plant.*

*Finally we learn that the astrality of plants is connected with
human bodily organs in ways that could in future be of widespread benefit to people's health. Echoes of this are to be found in
traditional medical practices in many parts of the world that
arose originally out of clairvoyant consciousness.*

Plants, minerals and creation

The Elohim placed the affairs of light and darkness in
charge of the Archai. While the Archai themselves are
active as Aeons, they make use of the Archangels, the
light-bearers who act from the periphery, for the deploy-
ment of their forces. That means that through the constellations of the light beings surrounding the earth, the
Archangels work out of cosmic space in such a way that
the great ordinances laid down by the Archai may be
carried into effect. They entrusted to the Archangels the
activity which has to stream to earth from outside so that
not only could plants develop but also an animal nature,
weaving its inward life of images and sensations.

Spiritual science can only speak in such a way that everything that belongs to the earth — that which someone looking at earth from space would find in human beings, animals, plants and stones — belongs to the whole of our earth. This means that we cannot look at planet earth as a dead rock formation but rather as something that is in itself a living whole, generating the nature of plants out of itself, just as the human being generates the structures of his skin, his sense organs, and the like. In other words, we cannot consider the earth without the plant cover that belongs to it.

Natural science likes to refer to the origins of all life — including plant life — lying in the lifeless, mineral element. This issue does not exist at all for the spiritual investigator, because the lower is never a precondition for the higher; on the contrary, the higher, the living, is always the precondition for the lower, the non-living.

Spiritual research shows how everything rocklike, mineral — from granite to the soil in the field — originated in a manner similar to what natural science says today about the origin of coal. Today coal is a mineral. What was it millions of years ago according to the concepts of natural science? Extensive, mighty forests covered large portions of the earth's surface; later they sank into the earth during shifts of the earth's crust and were then transformed chemically, and what we dig up today out of the depths of the earth are the plants that have become stone. If this is accepted today in relation to coal, it should not be considered too ridiculous if spiritual science, by its methods, comes to the conclusion that all rocks found on our earth have originated from plants. Thus the mineral is not the precondition for the plantlike, but rather the reverse is the case, the plantlike is the precondition for the mineral. Everything of a mineral nature is first something plantlike that hardens and then turns to stone.

Thus the earth was once of a plant nature, was a structure of plantlike being, and only developed the lifeless out of what was living, progressively hardening, turning to wood, turning to stone.[30]

The plant world between earth and sun

Just as every stone, every lifeless body, shows its relationship to the earth by being able to fall onto the earth, where it encounters resistance, so every plant shows its relationship to the earth by the direction of its stem, which is always aligned such that it passes through the centre of the earth. All stems of plants would cross at the earth's centre if we extended them to that point. This means that the earth is able to draw out of its centre all those radiating forces that allow the plants to arise.

The truth about the soul nature of the plant world is that it has the plants for its individual organs.

Altogether there are seven group souls — plant souls — belonging to the earth, and having the centre of their being in the centre of the earth. So it is not enough to conceive of the earth as a physical sphere; but we have to think of it as penetrated by seven spheres varying in size and all having in the earth's centre their own spiritual centre. And then these spiritual beings impel the plants out of the earth.[31]

The plant soul is not to be found in the single plant but has its most important point in the centre of the earth; that is where the root goes, for the root is that force in the plant which strives towards the most spiritual part of plant existence.

What our senses are for us, the plants are for the earth organism. But what perceives, what achieves consciousness, is the spiritual world streaming down from the sun to the earth. This spiritual world would not be able to achieve consciousness if it did not have its sense organs in the plants, mediating a self-consciousness just as our eyes and ears and nerves mediate our self-consciousness. Those beings who stream from the sun down to the earth, unfolding their spiritual activity, encounter throughout spring and summer the being that belongs to the earth itself. In this exchange the organs are formed through which the earth perceives those beings, for the plants do not perceive.

The spiritual entities that belong to earth activity and sun activity perceive through the plant organs, and these entities direct towards the centre of the earth all organs they need in order to unite them with the centre of the earth. Thus what we can see behind the plant cover are the spiritual entities that weave around the earth and have their organs in the plants.

If we study the leaf of a plant, we will discover that the

outer surface is actually a composite of many small, lenslike structures.

These light organs can be compared to a kind of eye but the plant does not see by means of them; rather the sun being looks through them to the earth being. These light organs mean that the leaves of the plant always have the tendency to place themselves perpendicularly to the sunlight.

We have the plant's second main orientation in the way that the plant surrenders itself to the sun's activity. The first orientation is that of the stem, through which the plants reveal themselves as belonging to the earth's self-consciousness; the second orientation is the one through which the plants express the earth's surrender to the activity of the sun beings.

Thus we must look to mother earth as to our great nourishing mother. In the plant cover we have the physiognomy of the plant spirit, and this makes us feel as though we are standing in soul and spirit. It is like gazing into the soul of the earth—just as we gaze into the eyes of another person—if we understand how it manifests its soul in the blossoms and leaves of the plant world.

This is what led Goethe to occupy himself with the plant world, to engage in an activity that consisted fundamentally of showing how the spirit is active in the plant world and how in the plant the leaf is formed out of the spirit in the most diverse forms. Goethe was delighted that the spirit in the plant shapes the leaves, rounds them, and also leads them to spiral around the stem.

Earth's seasonal and diurnal breathing processes

At the times when we concern ourselves in our souls with the great festivals of the year, it is good to recall before our inner eye, out of spiritual cosmic connections, the meaning of the year in terms of its festivals. And I should like to do this by setting before you how, under the influence of spiritual insights and over long ages, the year in terms of its festivals has gradually evolved out of the whole constitution of the earth. If we look at the earth and what happens on earth from such a perspective, we must make clear that we cannot conceive it as a mere conglomeration of minerals and rocks, as is done by modern mineralogy and geology. We must rather regard it as a living, ensouled organism, which creates the plants, the animals and the physical nature of the human being out of its own inner forces.

You know that the earth, with all the beings belonging to it, completely changes its aspect in the course of the year.

Today we intend to consider this cycle of the earth as a kind of mighty breathing process which it undertakes in relation to the surrounding cosmos. We can consider still other processes which take place on the earth and around it as breathing processes of a sort. We can even speak of a daily breathing process of the earth. But today we want to place before our inner eye the yearly cycle as a mighty breathing process of this kind, in which of course it is not air that is breathed in and out but rather those forces which are at work for example in vegetation, those forces which push the plants out of the earth in spring and which withdraw again into the earth in autumn.

Let us first look at the earth at the time of the winter solstice, in the last third of December.[32]

We can of course only consider one part of the earth in connection with this kind of breathing. We shall consider that part in which we ourselves dwell; the conditions are naturally reversed on the opposite side of the earth. We must picture the breathing of the earth in such a way that in one region there is exhalation and in the opposite region inhalation.

At the end of December, the earth has fully inhaled and is holding in itself the forces of which I just spoke. It has entirely sucked in its soul element.

At this time the earth has withdrawn its soul being into itself. Jesus is born on the earth at a time when it is alone with itself, is isolated as it were from the cosmos.

Now let us follow the earth further in its annual course up to the time of the spring equinox, the end of March.

The earth has just exhaled; the soul is still half within the earth, but it has exhaled; the streaming soul forces are pouring out into the cosmos. Whereas since December the force of the Christ impulse has been intimately bound up with the earth, with the soul element of the earth, we find that now this Christ impulse together with the outward flowing soul element is beginning to radiate around the earth. What flows out into spiritual cosmic space as the Christ-permeated soul of the earth must be met now by the force of the sunlight itself. While in December Christ withdrew the soul of the earth into its interior in order for it to be insulated from cosmic influences, now with the exhalation of the earth he begins to let his forces breathe out, to extend them to receive the forces of the sun which radiate towards him.

If we carry further our view of the earth's breathing process during the course of the year, we find the earth in yet a third condition in June. Now the earth has completely exhaled. The entire soul element of the earth has been poured forth into cosmic space; it is yielded up to cosmic space and is saturating itself with the forces of the sun and the stars. Christ, who is joined with this soul element of the earth, now unites his force also with the forces of the stars and the sun, flowing in the earth soul that is given over to the cosmos. It is St John's Day – midsummer. The earth has fully exhaled. In its outer physiognomy, with which it looks out into the universe, it reveals not its own inherent force, as it did at the time of the winter solstice; instead, the earth reveals on its surface the reflected forces of the stars, of the sun, of all that is in the cosmos outside it.

The old initiates, particularly those in the northern regions of Europe, felt the inner meaning and spirit of the time that is our June with greatest vitality. At this time they felt their own souls, along with the earth's soul, given over to the cosmic expanses. They felt themselves to be living not within the earthly realm, but rather in the cosmic spaces. Indeed they said the following: 'We live with our soul in the cosmic expanses. We live with the sun, we live with the stars.'

If we follow this breathing process still further we come finally to the stage that begins at the end of September. The exhaled forces begin their return movement; the earth begins once more to inhale. The soul of the earth which was poured out into the cosmos now draws back into the interior of the earth again. In their subconscious or in their clairvoyant impressions, human souls perceive this inhalation of the earth's soul element as processes within themselves.

Because the earth is a mirror of the cosmos in the summer, it is also opaque in its inner nature, impermeable to cosmic influences and therefore impermeable to the Christ impulse during the summer. At this time the Christ impulse has to live in the exhaled breath. The ahrimanic forces, however, establish themselves firmly in the earth. And when the human being returns once more with the forces which he has taken into his own soul through the earth's exhalation—including the forces of the Christ—he plunges into an earth which has been subject to the influence of Ahriman.

However, it is the case that since the last third of the nineteenth century, while the earth's breath is flowing back into the earth, the force of Michael comes to the aid of the human soul descending from spiritual heights, and does battle with the dragon, Ahriman.

This was already foreseen and prophesied by those in the ancient mysteries who understood the course of the year spiritually.

We can continually become aware of how in the earth's

environment there is not only that which comes directly from the sun but also that which partakes in the life of the earth beneath the surface of the soil. Those of you who have lived in the country will know how the farmers dig pits in the earth during winter and put their potatoes in them. Down there in the earth the potatoes last splendidly through the winter, which would not be the case if they were simply put in cellars. Why is this? Think of an area of the earth's surface. It absorbs the light and warmth of the sun that have streamed to it during the summer. The light and the warmth sink down, as it were, into the soil of the earth, so that in winter the summer is still there under the soil. During winter it is summer underneath the surface of the earth. And it is this summer under the surface of the earth in winter-time, that enables the roots of the plants to thrive. The seeds become roots and growth begins. So when we see a plant growing this year, it is actually being enabled to grow by the forces of last year's sun which have penetrated into the earth.

When therefore we are looking at the root of a plant, or even at parts of the leaves, we have before us in the plant the previous summer. It is only in the blossom that we have this year's summer, for the blossom is conjured up by the light and warmth of the present year's sun. In the sprouting and unfolding of the plant we still have the previous year and the present year comes to manifestation only in the blossom. Even the ovary at the centre of the blossom is a product of the winter — in reality, that is, of the previous summer. Only what surrounds the ovary

belongs to the present year. Thus the seasons interpenetrate. When the earth dons her winter raiment of
snow, beneath that raiment is the continuation of summer.

Mineral substances must emancipate themselves from
what is working immediately above the surface of the
earth if they wish to be exposed to the most distant cosmic
forces. In our age they can most easily do so — they can
most easily emancipate themselves from the earth's
immediate vicinity and come under the influence of the
most distant cosmic forces down inside the earth — in the
time between 15 January and 15 February, in the winter
season. This is the season when the strongest formative
forces of crystallization, the strongest forces of form, can
be developed for the mineral substances within the earth.
It is in the middle of the winter. The interior of the earth
then has the property of being least dependent on itself —
on its own mineral masses; it comes under the influence of
the crystal-forming forces that are there in the wide spaces
of the cosmos.

This then is the situation. Towards the end of January
the mineral substances of the earth have the greatest
longing to become crystalline, and the deeper we go into
the earth, the more they have this longing to become
purely crystalline within 'nature's household'. Plants at
this time are mostly left to themselves within the earth;
they are least exposed to the mineral substances. On the
other hand, for a certain time before and after this
period — and notably before it, when the minerals are on
the point of passing over into the crystalline element of

form and shape — then they are of the greatest importance; they ray out the forces that are particularly important for plant growth. Thus we may say that approximately in the months of November and December there is a point of time when what is under the surface of the earth becomes especially effective for plant growth.

Now a great distinction must be made between what I will call warmth night and warmth day. During warmth night, when we are not exposed to the sun being, when the earth being is left to itself and can emancipate itself from the influences of the cosmic sun being, the earth strives for form as the droplet takes on form when it can withdraw itself from the general force of gravitation. In warmth night the earth strives towards formation, towards crystallization. And what we experience every night is a continuous emergence of lines of forces striving towards crystallization, whereas during the day, under the influence of the being of the sun, there is a continual dissolving of this striving towards crystallization, a continual will to overcome form.

In the future we must be able to do a given experiment during the day and repeat it at a corresponding hour of the night, and we must have sensitive measuring instruments that will show us the difference in the way the process goes by day and by night. For by day those forces striving towards crystallization in the earth are not active in the process but they are at night. Forces arise that come from the cosmos in the night. And these cosmic forces that seek to crystallize the earth must be revealed in the phenomena. This opens a way of experimentation that will show once again the relationship of the earth to the cosmos.[33]

Trees and the astral environment of plants

The plant grows out of the ground. The root grows out of the seed. Let us take a tree: the stem grows up. This growth is very remarkable. This stem is really only formed because it lets sap mount from the earth and so the stem becomes hard.

What happens, in reality? The earthy, the solid, becomes fluid. And we have an earthy-fluid substance mounting there. Then the fluid evaporates and the solid remains behind: that is the wood.

You see, this sap which mounts up in the tree — let us call it wood-sap — is not created there but is already contained everywhere in the earth, so that the earth in this respect is really a great living being. This sap which mounts in the tree is really present in the whole earth, only in the earth it is something special. It becomes in the tree what we see there. In the earth it is in fact the sap which actually gives it life. For the earth is really a living being; and that which mounts in the tree is present in the whole earth and through it the earth lives. In the tree it loses its life-giving quality. It becomes merely a chemical; it has only chemical qualities.

Through the sap the plant is connected with the earth; the life-sap connects the plant with what circulates round the earth—with the airy-moist circumference of the earth. But the cambium brings the plant into connection with the stars, with what is above, and in such a way that within this cambium the form of the next plant develops. This passes over to the seeds and in this way the next plant is born, so that the stars indirectly through the cambium create the next plant.

It is really wonderful—a seed, a humble, modest little seed could only come into existence because the cambium imitates the whole plant; and this form which arises there in the cambium—a new plant form—this carries the power to the seed to develop through the forces of the earth into a new plant.

So it is with trees, and so too with the ordinary plants. When the rootlet is in the earth, the sprout shoots upwards. But it does not separate off the solid matter, does not make wood; it remains like a cabbage stalk. The leaves come out directly on the circumference in spirals, the cambium is formed directly in the interior, and the cambium takes everything back to the earth with it. In the annual plants the whole process occurs much more quickly. In the tree, only the hard parts are separated out, and not everything is destroyed. The same process occurs in ordinary plants, too, but is not carried so far as in trees.

As for the cambium, there the whole plant is sketched out from the stars. The wood sap rises and dies, then life again arises; and now comes the influence of the stars, so that from the thick, sticky cambium the new plant is sketched out. In the cambium one has a sketch, a sculptural activity. The stars model in it the complete plant form from the whole of the universe. So you see, we come from life to the spirit. What is modelled there is modelled from out of the cosmic spirit. The earth first gives up her life to the plant, the plant dies, the air environment along with its light once more gives it life, and the cosmic spirit implants the new plant form. This is preserved in the seed and grows again in the same way.

So that one sees in the growing plant how the plant world rises out of the earth, through death, to the living spirit.

To understand a tree, we must say: here is the thick tree-trunk (and in a sense the boughs and branches still belong to it). The real plant grows out of it. Leaves, flowers and fruit grow out of it; they are the real plant—rooted in the trunk and branches of the tree, as the herbaceous plants and cereals are rooted in the earth.

The plant which grows on the tree has lost its root. Relatively speaking, it is even separated from its root— only it is united with it, as it were, in a more etheric way. What I have sketched is actually there in the tree, as the cambium layer. That is how we must regard the roots of these plants that grow out of the tree; they are replaced by the cambium. Although the cambium does not look like roots, it is the living, growing layer, constantly forming new cells, so that the plant life of the tree grows out of it, just as the life of a herbaceous plant grows up above out of the root below.

The tree with its cambium or formative layer is actually

an extension of the earth realm; it has grown outwards into the airy regions. And having thus grown outwards into the air, it needs more inwardness, more intensity of life, than the earth otherwise has, than it has where the ordinary root is in it. Now we begin to understand the tree. In the first place, we understand it as a strange entity whose function is to separate the plants that grow upon it — stem, blossom and fruit — from their roots, uniting them only through the spirit, that is, through the etheric. We must learn to look with macrocosmic intelligence into the mysteries of growth. But it goes still further. For I now ask you to observe what happens through the fact that a tree comes into being. It is as follows.

What grows up there on the tree has a different plant nature in the air and outer warmth than that which grows in air and warmth immediately on the soil, unfolding the herbaceous plant that springs out of the earth directly. It is a different plant world for it is far more intimately related to the surrounding astrality. Down here, the astrality in air and warmth is expelled, so that the air and warmth may become mineral for the sake of the human being and animal. Look at a plant growing directly out of the soil. True, it is surrounded, enshrouded in an astral cloud. Up there, however, round about the tree, the astrality is far denser. Our trees are gatherings of astral substance; quite clearly, they are gatherers of astral substance.

For a great distance around, the tree makes the spiritual atmosphere inherently richer in astrality. The tree has a certain inner vitality or ethericity; it has a certain intensity of life.[34] Now the cambium damps down this life a little more, so that it becomes slightly more mineral. While up above a rich astrality arises all around the tree, the cambium works in such a way that inside the ethericity is poorer.

Within the tree arises poverty of etheric substance as compared to the plant. And as the cambium engenders a relative poverty of etheric substance in the tree, the root in its turn will be influenced. The roots of the tree become mineral — far more so than the roots of herbaceous plants. And the root, being more mineral, deprives the earthly soil of some of its ethericity. This makes the earthly soil rather more dead in the environment of the tree than it would be in the environment of a herbaceous plant.

What becomes very evident in the tree is present in a more delicate way throughout the whole plant world. In every plant there is a tendency to become treelike. In every plant, the root with its environment strives to let go the etheric substance, while that which grows upwards tends to draw in the astral more densely.

I have told you on several occasions that the plant form consists of the physical body and the etheric body belonging to it but that in its upward growth it extends its blossoms into the surrounding astrality; when we survey a bed of plants we find astrality spread out over the plants, astrality belonging to the plants. The single plant does not have an astral body; but the general astrality spread out over the surface of the earth, as the air is spread out physically, is nevertheless differentiated. What alights, shall we say, on a particular lily blossom out of the astral body of the earth has a different appearance from that which descends on a clover blossom. Here the general astrality differentiates itself.

This relationship between the whole terrestrial astrality and the carpet of plant life spread out over the earth also exists inwardly between the human astral body and its organs. In this sense, too, man is wholly a microcosm.

The relationship that exists between the general astrality of the earth and the entire plant life covering the earth is generally speaking a healthy one, and when one discovers the relations between the single plants and the human organs it will become possible to stimulate and to cure the organs from within by administering substances from the relevant plants. For when these plant substances are introduced into the human organism, the plant's relationship to the general astrality of the earth is brought in as well. If this relationship becomes blunted in the human organism, it receives a new stimulus in the human astral body as well when one applies the forces of the appropriate plant.[35] Here arises the possibility of establishing a plant system which corresponds to the human organism and which will still constitute a rational system of certain remedies for specific organic diseases.

4. Farms and the Realms of Nature

*The study of ecology has made us aware of the interconnected-
ness of the natural world, a fact underlined by many current
farming and environmental problems. Here, to begin with,
Steiner invites us to consider the farm as a microcosm of the
living earth, with the farm animal, notably the cow, depending
on the plant world and thus forming a link between the life of the
farm and the earth as a whole. It is in this context that the ideal of
self-sufficiency of input is stressed. It is explained why the dung
from the cow has such special properties and why animal manure
is different from that of humans. The cow is able to concentrate
astral forces within its digestive system because of the special
characteristics of horns and hoofs. Such insights about horns and
manure form the basis for a special enhancement of cow manure
(see Chapter 7, pp. 132–4).*

*We then consider the role of the earth's flying creatures,
pointing to their importance in spreading astral fertilizing
influences in the life of plants. In addition, the winged creatures
perform a task in the spiritualization of substance which com-
pletes a cycle of spiritual activity, enabling higher beings to
experience something of the work they have done on the earth. As
the diversity of species of all kinds diminishes we can only
wonder how this will play into the future vitality of living
processes on the earth.*

According to Steiner, the plant nature does not fall prey to disease as does that of animals and humans. Nevertheless, their living environment can be so out of balance that processes normally confined to the destruction of dying and dead organic materials become directed at living tissues. While lack of vitality through poor nutrition renders plants vulnerable to such influences, here Steiner mentions the over-emphasis of watery influence on the plant as a major problem. This arises from chemical agriculture and its link with readily soluble nutrients but also from prolonged dull and damp weather. Suggestions are offered for strengthening plants against such eventualities rather than the more common approach of attacking the pathogenic organism.

Animals and the farm individuality

A farm is true to its essential nature, in the best sense of the word, if it is conceived as a kind of individual entity in itself—a self-contained individuality. Every farm should approximate to this condition. This ideal cannot be absolutely attained, but it should be observed as far as possible. Whatever you need for agricultural production, you should try to possess it within the farm itself (including in the farm, needless to say, the due amount of cattle).

We shall see presently why this is the natural thing. So long as one does not regard things in their true essence but only in their outer material aspect, the question may justifiably arise: is it not a matter of indifference whether we get our cow dung from the vicinity or from our own farm?

But it is not so. Although these things may not be able to be strictly carried out, we do, nevertheless, need to have this ideal concept of the necessary self-contained nature of any farm if we wish to do things in a proper and natural way.

You will recognize the justice of this statement if, on the one hand, you consider the earth from which our farm arises, and, on the other hand, what works down into our earth from the universe beyond. Nowadays, people speak very abstractly of the influences which work on the earth from the surrounding universe. They are aware, no doubt, that the sun's light and warmth and all the meteorological processes connected with it are in a way related to the form and development of the vegetation that covers the soil. But present-day ideas can give no real information as to the exact relationships, because they do not penetrate to the realities involved. Let us consider, to begin with, the soil, which is the foundation of all agriculture.

The surface of the earth is generally regarded as mere mineral matter which might at best include some organic elements to the extent that there is formation of humus or that manure is added. In reality, however, the soil as such not only contains a certain life — a vegetative nature of its own — but an effective astral principle as well, a fact which not only fails to be taken into account today but is not even admitted. But we can go still further. We must observe that this inner life of the soil is different in summer and in winter. Here we are coming to a realm of knowledge, immensely significant for practical life, that is not even conceived in our time.

Taking our start from a study of the soil, we must indeed observe that the surface of the earth is a kind of organ in that organism which reveals itself throughout the growth of nature. The earth's surface is a real organ, which may be compared to the human diaphragm. We gain a right idea of these facts if we say: above the human diaphragm there are certain organs, notably, the head and the processes of breathing and circulation which work up into the head. Beneath it there are other organs.

If from this point of view we now compare the earth's surface with the human diaphragm, then we must say: in the entity with which we are here concerned, the head is beneath the surface of the earth, while we, with all the animals, are living in the creature's belly.[36] Whatever is above the earth belongs in truth to the intestines of the 'agricultural individuality', to coin the phrase. We, in our farm, are going about in the belly of the farm, and the plants themselves grow upwards in the belly of the farm. Indeed, we are dealing with an entity standing on its head. We only regard it rightly if we imagine it as standing on its head in comparison to the human being.

And now, to localize these influences, please observe the following. The activities above the earth are directly dependent on moon, Mercury and Venus supplementing and modifying the influences of the sun. The planets near the earth extend their influences to all that is above the earth's surface. On the other hand, the distant planets work upon all that is beneath the earth's surface, assisting those influences which the sun exercises from below the earth. Thus, so far as plant growth is concerned, we must look for the influences of the distant heavens beneath, and of the earth's immediate cosmic environment above the earth's surface.

All that works inwards from the far spaces of the cosmos to influence the growth of plants works not directly — not by direct radiation — but is first received by the earth; and the earth then rays it upwards again. We are talking not only about direct sunlight; we are also talking about the sunlight reflected by the moon. This sunlight reflected by the moon is quite ineffective when it shines onto the head of an animal. There it has no influence. (What I am now saying applies especially, however, to the embryonic life.) The light that is rayed back from the moon develops its greatest influence when it falls on the hind parts of the animal. Look at the skeleton formation of the hind parts; observe its peculiar relation to the head formation. Cultivate a sense of form to perceive this contrast — the attachment of the thighs, the formation of the outgoing parts of the digestive tract, in contrast to that which is formed as the opposite pole, from the head inwards. There, in the fore and hind parts of the animal, you have the true contrast of sun and moon.

Moreover you will find that the sun's influence goes as far as the heart and stops short just before the heart. Mars, Jupiter and Saturn are at work in the head and the blood-forming process. Then, from the heart backwards, the moon influence is supported by the Mercury and Venus forces. If therefore you turn the animal and stand it on its head, with the head stuck into the earth and the hind parts upwards, you have the position which the 'agricultural individuality' has invisibly.

Specific animals belong to specific regions of the earth. For the peculiar fact is that if you have the right amount of horses, cows and other animals in any given farm, these animals taken together will give just the amount of manure which you need for the farm itself, in order to add something more to what has already turned into chaos.

Indeed, if you have the right number of cows, horses, pigs, and so on, the individual proportion of admixture in the manure will also be correct. This is due to the fact that the animals will eat the right measure of what is provided for them by the growth of plants. They eat the right quantity of what the earth is able to provide. Hence in the course of their organic processes they bring forth just the amount of manure which needs to be given back again to the earth.

The following therefore applies. We cannot implement it in absolute terms, but in the ideal sense it is correct. If we are obliged to bring in manure from outside the farm, we should, properly speaking, only use it as a remedy — as medication for a farm that has already grown ill. The farm is only healthy inasmuch as it provides its own manure from its own stock. Naturally, this will necessitate our developing a proper science of the number of animals of a given sort that we need for a given kind of farm.

In the human being, as much as possible of the belly-manure is transformed into brain-manure, for the human being as you know carries his ego down onto the earth; in the animal, less so.[37] Therefore, more remains behind in the belly-manure in the animal and this is what we use for the manuring. Just because the animal itself does not reach up to the ego, more ego remains there potentially. Hence, animal and human manure are altogether different things. Animal manure still contains the ego in potential.

Picture how we manure the plant. We bring the manure from outside to the plant root. That is to say, we bring ego to the root of the plant. Down here you have the root; up there, the unfolding leaves and blossoms. There, through the intercourse with air, astrality unfolds—the astral principle is added—whereas down here, through intercourse with the manure, the ego potential of the plant develops.

Truly, the farm is a living organism. Above, in the air, it evolves its astrality. Fruit trees and woods by their very presence develop such astrality. And now when the animals feed on what is there above the earth, they in their turn develop the real ego forces. These they give off in the dung, and the same ego forces will cause the plant in turn to grow from the root in the direction of the force of gravity. Truly a wonderful interplay, but we must understand it stage by stage, progressively, increasingly.

To this extent your farm is a kind of individuality, and

you will gain the insight that you ought to keep your animals as much as possible within this mutual interaction.

There is an inner kinship of mammals to all that does not become tree and yet does not remain herblike—in other words, to the shrubs and bushes—the hazelnut, for instance. To improve our stock of mammals on a farm, we would do well to plant bushes or shrubs. By their presence they have a beneficial effect. See how they love the shrubs and bushes. They soon begin to take what they need. This has a wonderfully regulating effect on their remaining fodder.

You must know that the cosmic influences that are effective in a plant rise upwards from the interior of the earth. They are led upwards. Suppose a plant is especially rich in such cosmic influences. The animal that eats the plant will in its turn provide manure out of its whole organism on the basis of this fodder. Thereby it will provide the very manure that is most suited for the soil on which the plant is growing. Thus if you can read nature's language of forms, you will perceive all that is needed by the 'self-contained individuality' which a true farm or agricultural unit should be. However, the animal stock must also be included in it.

The cow, her horns and manure

Let us consider the ox or cow. I have frequently spoken of the pleasure to be gained from watching a herd of cattle

lying replete and satisfied in a meadow, and from observing the process of digestion which here again comes to
expression in the position of the body, in the expression of
the eyes, in every movement. Make the opportunity to
observe a cow lying in the meadow and its reaction when
a noise comes from one direction or another. It is really
marvellous to see how the animal raises its head, how in
this lifting there lies the feeling that it is all heaviness, that
it is not easy for a cow to lift its head, and there is something rather special going on.

The cow is the animal of digestion.[38] It is, moreover, the
animal which accomplishes digestion in such a way that
there lies in its digestive processes the earthly reflection of
something that actually lies outside the earth; its whole
digestive process is permeated with an astrality which
reflects the entire cosmos in a wonderful, light-filled way.
There is a whole world in this astral organism of the cow,
but everything is based on gravity, everything is so
organized that the earth's gravity works there. You have
only to consider that a cow is obliged to consume about an
eighth of its weight in food each day. The human being
can be satisfied with a fortieth part and remain healthy.
Thus the cow needs earth's gravity in order to fully meet
the needs of its organism. This organism is designed for
the gravity of matter. Every day the cow must metabolize
an eighth of her weight. This binds the cow with its
material substance to the earth; yet through its astrality it
is at the same time an image of the heights of the cosmos.
This is why the cow is an object of so much veneration for

those who follow the Hindu religion. The Hindu says to himself: the cow lives here on the earth; but through this fact it creates in physical matter, subject to gravity, an image of something that lies outside the earth.

Have you ever thought why cows have horns, or why certain animals have antlers? It is a most important question, and what ordinary science says about it is as a rule one-sided and superficial. Let us then try to answer the question: why do cows have horns? An organic or living entity need not only have streams of forces flowing outwards, it can also have streams of forces flowing inwards.

The cow has proper horns and hoofs. What happens at the places where the horns grow and the hoofs? A locality is formed which sends the streams inwards with more than usual intensity. In this locality the outer is strongly shut off; there is no communication through permeable skin or hair. The openings which otherwise allow the streams to pass outwards are completely closed. For this reason the horn is connected with the entire way that the animal is shaped.

The cow has horns in order to send into itself the formative astral and etheric forces, which, pressing inwards, are meant to penetrate right into the digestive organism. Precisely through the radiating forces from horns and hoofs, much work arises in the digestive organism itself.

Thus in the horn you have something well adapted by its inherent nature to ray back the living and astral properties into the inner life. In the horn you have something radiating life—indeed, even radiating astrality. If you could crawl about inside the living body of a cow — if you were there inside the belly of the cow — you would smell how the astral life and living vitality pours inwards from the horns. And the same applies to the hoofs.

What is farmyard manure? It is what entered as outer food into the animal, and was received and assimilated by the organism up to a certain point. It gave occasion for the development of dynamic forces and influences in the organism, but it was not primarily used to enrich the organism with material substance. On the contrary, it was excreted. Nevertheless, it has been inside the organism and has thus been permeated with an astral and etheric content. In the astral it has been permeated with the nitrogen-carrying forces, and in the etheric with oxygen-carrying forces. The mass that emerges as dung is permeated with all this. Imagine now: we take this mass and give it over to the earth.

What we are actually doing is to give the earth something etheric and astral which has its existence by rights inside the belly of the animal and there engenders forces of a plantlike nature. For the forces we engender in our digestive tract are of a plantlike nature. We ought to be very thankful that the dung remains over at all; for it carries astral and etheric contents from the interior of the organs out into the open. The astral and etheric adheres to it. We only have to preserve it and use it in the proper way.

In dung, therefore, we have before us something etheric and astral. For this reason it has a life-giving and also astralizing influence upon the soil, and, what is more, in the earth element itself — not only in the watery but notably in the earthly element. It has the force to overcome what is inorganic in the earthly element.

The mission of birds and insects

The fully developed insect lives and moves by virtue of the rich astrality which is wafted through the tree-tops.

Take, on the other hand, what becomes poorer in etheric substance down below in the soil. That which is poorer in etheric substance down below works through the larvae. Thus, if the earth had no trees, there would be no insects on the earth. The trees make it possible for the insects to exist. The insects fluttering around the parts of the tree that are above the earth — fluttering around the woods and forests as a whole — they have their very life through the existence of the woods. Their larvae, too, live by the very existence of the woods.

A wonderful fact emerges here: certain of these sub-terrestrial creatures develop the faculty to regulate the etheric vitality within the soil whenever it becomes too great. If the soil is tending to become too strongly living — if ever its livingness grows rampant — these subterranean animals see to it that the over-intense vitality is released. Thus they become wonderful regulators, safety-valves for the vitality inside the earth. These golden creatures — for they are of the greatest value to the earth — are none other than the earthworms.

Study the earthworm—how it lives together with the soil. These worms are wonderful creatures; they leave to the earth precisely as much etheric substance as it needs for plant growth. There under the earth you have the earthworms and similar creatures—distantly reminiscent of the larvae.

Now there is again a distant similarity between certain animals and the fully evolved, i.e., the winged insect world. These animals are the birds. In the course of evolution a wonderful thing has taken place between the insects and the birds. I will describe it in a picture. The insects said one day: 'We do not feel quite strong enough to work the astrality which sparkles and sprays around the trees. We therefore, for our part, will use the treeing tendency of other plants; there we will flutter about, and to you birds we will leave the astrality that surrounds the trees.' So there came about a regular division of labour between the bird world and the butterfly world, and now the two together work most wonderfully.

These winged creatures, each and all, provide for a proper distribution of astrality wherever it is needed on the surface of the earth or in the air. Remove these winged creatures, and the astrality would fail to deliver its true service; and you would soon detect it in a kind of stunting of the vegetation. For the two things belong together—the winged animals, and that which grows out of the earth into the air. Fundamentally, the one is unthinkable without the other. Hence the farmer should also be careful to let the insects and birds flutter around in the right way.

The farmer himself should have some understanding of the care of birds and insects. For in great nature everything, but everything is connected.

It is also true that when bees seek out honey nectar in a certain region, they remove it from the plants. But they take it away from the plants that we need for other purposes, such as for fruit and so forth. The strange thing is that fruit trees and similar plants thrive better in regions where there is apiculture than in regions where there is not.[39] When the bees remove the honey nectar from the plants, nature does not look idly on but creates even more such fruitful plants. So it is that the human being derives benefits not only from the honey the bees provide but also from what is offered by the plants that bees have visited. This is an important law, into which you can gain deep insight.

If one looks at a butterfly, or indeed any insect, from the stage of the egg to when it is fluttering away, it is the plant raised up into the air, fashioned in the air by the cosmos.[40] If one looks at a plant, it is the butterfly held in fetters below. The egg is claimed by the earth. The caterpillar is metamorphosed into leaf formation. The chrysalis formation is metamorphosed into what is contracted in the plant. And then the same principle that unfolds to produce the butterfly develops into the flower in the plant. Small wonder that such an intimate relationship exists between the world of the butterflies, the insect world in general, and the world of plants. For in truth the spiritual beings that underlie the insects, the butterflies, must say to themselves: 'Down here are our relatives; we must maintain allegiance with them, unite ourselves with them in the enjoyment of their fluids, and so on. They are our brothers who have been metamorphosed down into the domain of the earth, who have become fettered to the earthly.' And in their turn the spirits who ensoul the plants can look up to the butterflies and say: 'These are the heavenly relatives of the plant on earth.'

It is a unique experience to see an insect poised on a plant and at the same time to see how astrality holds sway above the blossom. Here the plant is striving away from the earthly. The plant's longing for the heavenly holds sway above the iridescent petals of the flower. The plant cannot of itself satisfy this longing. Thus there radiates towards it from the cosmos what is of the nature of the butterfly. In beholding this the plant realizes the satisfaction of its own desires. And this is the wonderful relationship existing in the environment of the earth, namely, that the longings of the plant world are assuaged in looking up to the insects, in particular the world of the butterflies. What the blossoming flower longs for, as it radiates its colour out into cosmic space, becomes for it something like known fulfilment when the butterfly approaches it with its shimmer of colours. Longing that makes warmth radiate outwards, satisfaction streaming in from the heavens—this is the interplay between the world of the flowering plants and the world of the butterflies. This is what we should see in the environment of the earth.

We said of the bird that at its death it can carry

spiritualized earth substance into the spiritual world, and that thereby, as a bird, it has the task in cosmic existence of spiritualizing earthly matter, thus being able to accomplish what cannot be done by the human being. Human beings have earth matter in their heads that has also been spiritualized to some degree, but they cannot take this earthly matter into the world in which they live between death and a new birth for they would continually have to endure unspeakable, unbearable, devastating pain if they were to carry this spiritualized earth matter into the spiritual world.

The bird world can do this, so that a connection is actually created between what is earthly and what is outside the earth. Earthly matter is gradually transformed into spirit, and the birds have the task of transferring this spiritualized earthly matter to the universe. One can actually say that when the earth reaches the end of its existence, this earth matter will have been spiritualized, and that the birds have their place in the whole system of earthly existence for the purpose of taking this spiritualized earth matter back into spirit land.

It is somewhat different with butterflies. The butterfly spiritualizes earthly matter to an even greater degree than the bird. The bird after all is much closer to the earth than the butterfly. Because the butterfly never actually leaves the region of the sun, it is in a position to spiritualize its matter to such a degree that it does not, like the bird, have to await its death, but even in life is continually restoring spiritualized matter to the cosmic environment of the earth.

Just think of the magnificence of all this in the whole cosmic system! Picture the earth with the world of the butterflies fluttering around it in its infinite variety, continually sending out into cosmic space the spiritualized earthly matter which this butterfly world yields up to the cosmos! Then, with such knowledge, we can contemplate the region of the butterfly world which encircles the earth with totally different feelings.

Fungi and plant diseases

Just as coniferous forests are intimately related to the birds, and bushes to the mammals, so again all that is mushroom, or fungus-like, has an intimate relation to the lower animal world — to the bacteria and suchlike creatures, and notably the harmful parasites. The harmful parasites go together with the mushrooms or fungi; indeed they develop wherever the fungi appear scattered and dispersed.

Thus there arise the well-known plant diseases and harmful growths on a coarser and larger scale. If now we have not only woods but meadows in the vicinity of the farm, these meadows will be very useful, inasmuch as they provide good soil for mushrooms and toadstools; and we should see to it that the soil of the meadow is well planted with such growths. If there is a meadow rich in mushrooms near the farm — it need not even be very large — the mushrooms, being akin to the bacteria and other parasitic creatures, will keep them away from everywhere else. For the mushrooms and toadstools, more than the other plants, tend to hold together with these creatures.

So we must look for a due distribution of wood and forest, orchard and shrubbery, as well as meadowlands with their natural growth of mushrooms. This is the very essence of good farming, and we shall achieve far more by such means, even if we reduce to some extent the surface available for tillage.

It is no true economy to exploit the surface of the earth to such an extent as to rid ourselves of all the things I have mentioned here in the hope of increasing our crops. Your large plantations will become worse in quality, and this will more than outweigh the extra amount you gain by increasing your tilled acreage at the cost of these other things.

It only remains for us to consider so-called plant diseases. Properly speaking, we cannot really say 'plant diseases'. The rather abnormal processes which occur are not diseases in the same sense as in animal diseases. They are not at all the same kind of process as in human diseases. Properly speaking, disease is not possible without the presence of an astral body. In an animal or human being, the astral body is connected with the physical through the etheric. The astral body may be connected more intensely with the physical (or with any one of its organs) than it should normally be. In such a case, the etheric body fails to provide a sufficient cushioning or 'padding' and the astral body drives into the physical too strongly. It is under these conditions that most of our illnesses arise.

Now the plant has no real astral body. Hence the specific way of being ill which can occur in the animal and in the human being does not occur in the plant. We must be well aware of this fact. Thus we must first gain an insight into the question: what is it that can bring about illness of plants?

You have seen from my descriptions how the earth in the plant's environment has an inherent life of its own. With all this life in the earth manifold forces of growth and faint suggestions of reproductive forces are present all around the plant. Moreover, there is all that which is working in the earth under the influence of the full moon forces, mediated by the water. Here is a wealth of significant relationships.

You have the earth, and you have the moon. The moon, letting its radiation pour into the earth, brings it to life to some extent, awakens etheric flows within the earth. It does so more easily when the earth is saturated with water, and with greater difficulty when the earth is dry. You must remember, the water is only a mediator. It is the earth itself—the solid, mineral element—which must be made alive. The water, too, is mineral. There is of course no hard-and-fast line. Thus we must have the lunar influences in the soil.

The moon influences in the soil can become too strong. This can happen in a very simple way. You need only call to mind a thoroughly wet winter, followed by a thoroughly wet spring. Then the moon forces will enter the earth too strongly. The earth will become too much alive.

If the moon imparts precisely the right vitality to the earth, this vitality will work on and upwards till the seed develops. Let us assume now that the moon influence is too strong; the earth is too much vitalized. Then it will work too strongly from below upwards. What should only occur at the time of seed formation will occur at an earlier stage. Precisely when it is too strong, it will be insufficient to reach to the top. Through its very intensity, it will exhaust itself to a greater extent in the lower regions. As a result, seed formation will have insufficient strength.

The seed receives something of dying life into itself, and through this dying life there arises above the soil — above the primary level of the earth — a secondary level. Although it is not earth, the same effects are there — above the proper level — and, as a consequence, the seed (the upper part of the plant) becomes a kind of soil for other organisms. Parasites and fungoid growths arise. Thus we see the forming of mildew, blight, rust, and similar diseases. What, then, should we do?

We must somehow relieve the earth of the excessive moon force that is in it. We need only perceive what works in the earth so as to deprive the water of its mediating power, so as to lend the earth more 'earthiness' and prevent it from absorbing the excessive moon influences through the water it contains. We now prepare a kind of tea or decoction — a concentrated decoction of *Equisetum arvense* (horsetail). This we dilute, and sprinkle as liquid manure over the fields, wherever we need it — wherever we want to combat rust or similar plant diseases. Very small quantities are sufficient — a homoeopathic dose is quite enough.[41]

Now we may be concerned with the occurrence of plant diseases. In healing, we must proceed not from the histological or microscopic diagnosis, but from the great universal connections. And so it is in relation to plant nature. This is simpler than animal or human nature. For the plant world, we can apply a kind of universal remedy.

A large number of plant diseases can be removed as soon as we observe them, by an improvement in manuring; that is, by the following methods.

We must introduce calcium into the soil with the manure. But it is no use to introduce the calcium into the soil by means that avoid the living sphere. To have a healing effect, the calcium must remain within the realm of life. Ordinary lime or the like is of no use in this respect.

Now there is a plant containing plenty of calcium. I refer to the oak — notably, the bark of the oak, which represents an intermediate product between plant nature and living earth nature. As it appears in this connection, the calcium structure in the bark of the oak is ideal.[42]

Now calcium restores order when the etheric body is working too strongly, thereby liberating the influences of the astral body. So it is with all limestone. If we want uncontrolled etheric development of whatever kind to be reduced in a controlled manner—so that its reduction is beautiful and regular and does not give rise to shocks in the organism—then we must use calcium in the structure in which we find it in the bark of the oak.

5. Bringing the Chemical Elements to Life

In order to break loose from the conventional view of physical matter one has to take into account the fundamental influence of cosmic forces and the particular conditions on earth which have brought about matter as we experience it. Thus the atom – a true image of the cosmos – is seen to reflect on the most microscopic scale an interaction of matter and energy, which, as it turns out, represents a projection of opposing spiritual powers.

Plant life is directly affected by the planetary system and its motions and in this chapter, without covering more than a few aspects of plant morphology, we see how complex an interplay there is. Whereas we can view the outer cosmos as raying forces into our solar system – a harmony perhaps – the planetary bodies work with these forces to create the rhythms which affect the growth of organisms. The inner and outer planets together with sun and moon influence life in different ways and their forces connect with categories of earthly substances represented here by silicon and calcium. To a large extent silicon represents a cosmic sensing and giving while calcium is concerned with receiving and with the desire for spiritual life to incarnate.

Finally, the earthly elements which comprise much of the weight of organisms have also their cosmic significance and Steiner presents a picture of how each plays its part in the wholeness of nature. In scientific terms this is a huge contribution to the spiritualization of chemistry and it significantly alters our feelings about the nature of substance and how we should approach the growth of crops and animals.

The nature of the atom

What the stars, like giants, do in presenting their many-sided relationships in earthly processes is given expression by the dwarves of atoms and molecules. Indeed, we should know that when we represent a material, earthly process or perform calculations on it, we are dealing with nothing other than an image of extraterrestrial, of cosmic interactions.

Let us hold on to the fact that there are those whose speculations are mainly concerned with matter; they imagine that the world consists of atoms. How does this view compare with what spiritual science has to say? Certainly natural physical phenomena do lead us back to atoms, but what are these atoms? They reveal what they are at the moment the very first stage of spiritual perception has been attained. At the stage of imaginative perception atoms reveal what they truly are. Those who speculate on matter come to the conclusion that space is empty and atoms whirl around in this empty space. Atoms are supposed to be the most solid entities in existence. That is simply not the case; the whole issue is based on illusion. To imaginative cognition atoms are revealed as bubbles and the reality is where the empty space is supposed to be. Atoms are blown up bubbles. In other words, in contrast to what surrounds them they are nothing. You know that where bubbles are seen in soda-water there is no water. Atoms are bubbles in that sense; where they are the space is hollow, nothing is there. And yet it is possible to push against it; impact occurs precisely because, in pushing against hollowness, an effect is produced.[43]

Atoms are empty — and yet again not empty. There is, after all, something within these bubbles. And what is it? This is something about which I have already spoken — what exists within the atom bubbles is ahrimanic substance. Ahriman is there.[44] The whole system of atoms consists of ahrimanic substance. As you see, this is a considerable metamorphosis of the ideas entertained by those who theorize about matter. Where in space they see something material we see the presence of Ahriman. Force is another concept. Here again the very first stage of spiritual cognition shows that where force is supposed to be active there is in fact nothing. But where the force is thought not to be, there something is at work. It is exactly as if two people walked side by side and were observed by a third person. He looks towards them and, as they are walking a little apart, he looks between them and describes not the people but the space between them. He is concerned not with the two people but the emptiness between them. That is the way those who theorize about force are looking at what is between the reality.

Physicists draw lines to depict currents of force. But where the force is supposed to be there is in fact nothing, whereas all around there is something. There is Lucifer, the luciferic element. If we want to depict what corresponds to actual reality we must place the luciferic element where force is placed by those who theorize about it.

What can be described as force and matter are really depicted by Lucifer and Ahriman. You may say: this is dreadful! It is not dreadful for as I have often emphasized, Lucifer and Ahriman are only dreadful when they are not balanced against each other. In mutual balance they serve the wise guidance of the cosmos. When Lucifer is placed on one side of the scales and Ahriman on the opposite side, the balance between them must be achieved. It is a balance for which we must constantly strive.

Planetary influences on earthly life

We shall never understand plant life unless we bear in mind that everything which happens on the earth is but a reflection of what is taking place in the cosmos. For the human being this fact is only masked because he has emancipated himself; he only bears the inner rhythms in himself. To the plant world, however, it applies in the highest degree.

The earth is surrounded in the heavens first by the moon and then by the other planets of our planetary system. In an old instinctive science which reckoned the sun among the planets, they had this sequence: moon, Mercury, Venus, sun, Mars, Jupiter, Saturn.

If you follow the process of plant growth as it moves upwards, away from the earthly element, the first thing to become aware of is the spiral path of development of both leaves and flowers. The plant's formative forces trace a spiral of sorts around the stem. This spiral path cannot be deduced from inner forces of tension within the plant but must be attributed to extratelluric influences and especially to the effects of the apparent path of the sun. The sun force would take possession of plants completely and make them continue into infinity if it, in turn, were not counteracted by the forces of the so-called outer planets.

We must count Mars, Jupiter and Saturn as belonging to the outer planets. The forces of the outer planets cause the force directed upwards to retreat. They bring about the development of flowers and fruit by restraining what would otherwise be expressed only in the spiral of the leaves. If you study plant growth above the leaves, you must attribute its origin to the forces that come about as the result of the sun working together with Mars, Jupiter and Saturn.

Not only do these two elements work together, however, but they are also counteracted by what comes from the moon, in particular, and also from the so-called inner planets, Mercury and Venus. Mercury, Venus and the moon engender the downward, earth-directed tendency in the plant; their most characteristic expression lies in the development of roots. Everything that appears earthly is actually simultaneously influenced by the moon and the inner planets. You might say that the plant is an expression of our entire solar system.

What do we know of the moon in ordinary life? We know that it receives the rays of the sun upon its surface and reflects them to the earth. We see the rays of the sun reflected — we catch them with our eyes — and the earth, too, of course, receives these rays from the moon. It is the rays of the sun which are thus reflected, but of course the moon permeates them with its own forces. They come to the earth as lunar forces, and so they have done ever since the moon separated from the earth.

Now in the cosmos it is just this lunar force which strengthens and intensifies all that is earthly. Indeed, when the moon was united with the earth, the earth itself was far more alive, fruitful, inherently fertile. When the moon was still one with the earth there was nothing so mineral as we have today. Even now, after its severance, the moon works so as to intensify the normal vitality of the earth, which is still just enough to bring about the growth in living creatures. The moon intensifies it, thus enhancing the growth process to the point of reproduction.[45]

People commonly imagine that the moon merely receives the sun's rays and throws them down onto the earth. But that is not the only thing that comes to the earth.

With the moon's rays the whole reflected cosmos comes to the earth. All influences that pour onto the moon are rayed back again. Thus the whole starry heavens — though we may not be able to prove it by the customary physical methods of today — are rayed back onto the earth by the moon. It is indeed a strong and powerfully organizing cosmic force which the moon rays down into the plant, so that the seeding process of the plant may also be assisted; so that the force of growth may be enhanced into the force of reproduction.

The green leaves in their shape and thickness, and in their greenness too, carry an earthly element, but they would not be green unless the cosmic force of the sun were also living in them. This applies even more so when you come to the colourful flowers; in them live not only the cosmic forces of the sun, but also the supplementary forces that the sun forces receive from the distant planets—Mars, Jupiter and Saturn. This is how we must look at all plant growth. Then, when we contemplate the rose, we shall see the forces of Mars in its red colour. Or when we look at the yellow sunflower, it is not quite right to call it that because it is given that name on account of its form; as to its yellowness, it should really be named the Jupiter flower. For the force of Jupiter, supplementing the cosmic force of the sun, brings forth the white or yellow colour in flowers. And when we consider chicory, we will discover in its bluish colour the influence of Saturn, supplementing that of the sun. Thus we can recognize Mars in the red flower, Jupiter in yellow or white, Saturn in blue, while in the green leaf we see essentially the sun itself. But what thus shines out in the colouring of the flower works as a force most strongly in the root. For the forces that live and abound in the distant planets are working, as we have seen, down there below within the earthly soil.

That is how it is. Suppose we pull a plant out of the earth. Down below we have the root. In the root there is cosmic nature, whereas in the flower there is mostly earthly nature, the cosmic only being present in the delicate quality of the colouring and shading. If, on the other hand, earthly nature is to live strongly in the root, it must express its form. For the plant always takes its shape from that which can arise within the earthly realm. That which expands the form is earthly. Therefore cosmic roots are those that are more or less single in form. In highly ramified roots we have a working of earthly nature downwards into the soil, while in colour we have a working-upward of cosmic nature into the flower.

The sun quality is in the middle between the two. The sun nature lives most of all in the green leaf, in the mutual interplay between the flower and the root and all that is between them. The sun quality is really that which is related as a 'diaphragm' with the surface of the earth. The cosmic is associated with the interior of the earth and works upwards into the upper parts of the plant. The earthly, which is localized above the surface of the earth, works downwards, being carried down into the plant with the help of the limestone element.

Silica, lime and clay

Turning our attention to earthly life on a large scale, the first fact for us to take into account is this. The greatest imaginable part is played in this earthly life by all that which we may call the life of the siliceous substance in the world. You will find siliceous substance, for example, in the beautiful mineral quartz, enclosed in the form of a prism and pyramid; you will find the siliceous substance, combined with oxygen, in the crystals of quartz.

Now what does this silicon do? Let us assume that we only had half as much silicon in our earthly environment. In that case our plants would all have more or less pyramidal forms. On the other hand we find another kind of substance, which occurs everywhere throughout the earth, although it is not so widespread as the siliceous element. I mean the chalk or limestone substances and all that is akin to these — limestone, potash, sodium substances. Again, if these were present to a lesser extent, we would have plants with very thin stems — plants, to a large extent, with twining stems; they would all become like creepers. Plant life in the form in which we see it today can only thrive in the equilibrium and cooperation of the two forces.

Now we can go still farther. Everything that lives in siliceous nature contains forces which come not from the earth but from the outer planets, the planets beyond the sun — Mars, Jupiter and Saturn. That which proceeds from these distant planets influences the earth's plant and animal life via the siliceous and similar substances. On the other hand, from all that is represented by the planets near the earth — moon, Mercury and Venus — forces work via limestone and similar substances. Thus we may say that siliceous and limestone influences are working in every tilled field.

Everything connected with the inner force of reproduction and growth—everything that contributes to the sequence of generations in the plants—works through those forces which come down from the cosmos to the earth from moon, Venus and Mercury, via limestone.

On the other hand, when plants become foodstuffs for animal and the human being, then Mars, Jupiter and Saturn, working via silicon, are involved in the process. Siliceous nature opens the plant being to the wide spaces of the universe and awakens the senses of the plant being in such a way as to receive from all quarters of the universe the forces that are moulded by these distant planets.

It is through the sand, with its siliceous content, that the etheric and chemically active elements of the soil are infused into the earth. These influences then take effect as they ray upwards again from the earth.

What the plant roots experience in the soil depends in no small measure on the extent to which the cosmic life and cosmic chemistry are seized and held by means of the stones and the rock, which may well be at a considerable depth beneath the surface.

All that is thus connected, by way of silica, with the roots must also be able to be led upwards through the plant. It must flow upwards. There must be constant interaction between what is drawn in from the cosmos by the silicon and what takes place—forgive me!—in the 'belly' up above; for by the latter process the 'head' beneath must be supplied with what it needs. The 'head' is supplied out of the cosmos, but it must also be in mutual interaction with what is going on in the 'belly' above the earth's surface.[46] In a word, that which flows down from the cosmos and is caught up beneath the surface must be able to flow upwards again. And this is the purpose served by the clay in the soil. Everything in the nature of clay is in reality a means of transport for the influences of cosmic entities within the soil, to carry them upwards again from below.

But this upward flow of the cosmic influences is not all. There is also the other process, which I may call the terrestrial or earthly — that process which is going on in the 'belly' and which depends on a kind of external 'digestion'. For plant growth, in effect all that goes on through summer and winter in the air above the earth is essentially a kind of digestion. All that is thus taking place through a kind of digestive process must in its turn be drawn downwards into the soil. Thus a true mutual interaction will arise with all the forces and fine homoeopathic substances which are engendered by the water and air above the earth. All this is drawn down into the soil by the greater or lesser limestone content of the soil. The limestone content of the soil itself and the distribution of limestone substances in homoeopathic dilution immediately above the soil — all this is there to carry into the soil the immediate terrestrial process.

If people believe that they can only see the silica where it has a hard mineral outline, they are mistaken. In homoeopathic proportions, the siliceous principle is everywhere around us; moreover it rests in itself—it makes no claims. Limestone claims everything; the silicon principle claims nothing for itself. It is like our own sense organs. They too do not perceive themselves, but that which is outside them. Silica is the universal sense within the earthly realm, limestone the universal craving; and clay mediates between the two. Clay stands rather nearer to silica, but it still mediates towards the limestone.[47]

The elements of organic substance

One of the most important questions in agriculture is that of the significance of nitrogen—its influence on all farm production.

Nitrogen as it works in nature has four sisters, in a manner of speaking, whose working we must learn to know at the same time if we want to understand the functions and significance of nitrogen itself in nature's so-called household. The four sisters of nitrogen are those that are united with it in plant and animal protein in a way that is not yet clear to the external science of today. I mean carbon, oxygen, hydrogen and sulphur.

In order to know the full significance of protein, it is not sufficient to enumerate as its main ingredients hydrogen, oxygen, nitrogen and carbon. We must include another substance of the profoundest importance for protein, and that is sulphur. Sulphur in protein is the very element which acts as mediator between the spiritual that is spread throughout the universe—the formative power of the spiritual—and the physical.

We can indeed say that anyone who wants to trace the tracks which the spiritual marks out in the material world must follow the activity of sulphur. Though this activity appears less obvious than that of other substances, it is nevertheless of great importance; for it is along the paths of sulphur that the spiritual affects the physical domain of nature. Sulphur is actually the carrier of the spiritual.

Let us begin with carbon.

What is known about carbon nowadays is very little when you consider its infinite significance in the universe. The time is not so very long ago—only a few centuries— when this black fellow, carbon, was so highly esteemed as to be called by a very noble name. They called it the stone of the wise—the Philosopher's Stone.

The amorphous, formless substance which we see as coal or carbon proves to be only the last excrescence, the corpse of that which coal or carbon truly is in nature's household.

Carbon, in effect, is the bearer of all the creatively formative processes in nature. Whatever in nature is formed and shaped—be it the form of the plant persisting for a comparatively short time or the eternally changing configuration of the animal body—carbon is everywhere the great sculptor. Wherever we find it in full action and inner mobility, it bears within it the creative and formative cosmic pictures, the sublime cosmic imaginations, out of which all that is formed in nature must ultimately proceed.

There is a hidden sculptor in carbon, and this sculptor — building the manifold forms that are created in nature — makes use of sulphur in the process. To see carbon as it works in nature, we must see the spirit activity of the wide universe, making itself moist so-to-speak with sulphur, and working as a sculptor — building with the help of carbon the firmer and more well-defined form of the plant, or again, building the form in the human being which disappears again the very moment it comes into being.

For it is in this way that the human being does not turn into a plant but is a human being. He has the faculty time and again to destroy the form as soon as it arises; for he excretes the carbon, bound to oxygen, as carbon dioxide. Carbon in the human body would form us too stiffly and firmly — it would stiffen our form like a palm. Carbon is constantly about to make us stiff and firm in this way, and for this precise reason our breathing must constantly dismantle what carbon builds. Our breathing tears the carbon out of its rigidity, unites it with the oxygen and carries it outwards. So we are formed in the mobility which we as human beings need. In plants, the carbon is present in a very different way. To a certain degree it is fastened — even in annual plants — in a firm configuration.

It is on the paths of this carbon — moistened with sulphur — that the ego of the human being moves through the blood. So in a manner of speaking the ego of the universe lives via the sulphur in the carbon as it forms itself and ever again dissolves such form.

To a certain extent, the carbon in the human being and animal masks its native power of configuration. It finds a pillar of support in the configurative forces of limestone and silicon. Limestone gives it the earthly, silicon the cosmic formative power. Carbon, therefore, in the human being — and in the animal — does not declare itself exclusively responsible, but seeks support in the formative activities of limestone and silicon.

Carbon is the true creator of form in all plants; it is carbon that forms the structure or scaffolding. But in the course of Earth evolution this has been made difficult for carbon. It can form the plants if water is beneath it. Then it is equal to the task. But when limestone is there below, the limestone disturbs it. Therefore it allies itself to silica. Silica and carbon together — in union with clay, once again — create the forms. They do so in alliance because the resistance of the limestone must be overcome.

Now whether it be the human being or any other living thing, a living being must always be penetrated by an etheric element — for the etheric is the true bearer of life, as we have often emphasized. Therefore the carbon structure of a living entity must, in turn, be permeated by an etheric element. The latter will either stay still — holding fast to the structure — or it will be involved in a greater or lesser fluctuating movement. In either case, the etheric element must be spread out wherever the structure is. Now this etheric element, if it remained alone, could certainly not exist as such within our physical earth world. It would always slide through into the void. It could not hold what it must take hold of in the physical earth world if it had not a physical carrier. This, after all, is the specific character of what we have here on earth, that the spiritual must always have a physical carrier.

What then is the physical carrier of that spiritual element which works in the etheric? The physical element which with the help of sulphur carries the influences of the universal etheric into the physical is none other than oxygen.[48] Only now does the breathing process reveal its meaning. In breathing we absorb oxygen in which the lowest of the supersensory elements, the etheric, lives.

Inside us, the oxygen is not the same as it is where it surrounds us externally. Within us, it is living oxygen and in like manner it becomes living oxygen the moment it passes from the atmosphere we breathe into the soil of the earth. Although it does not live there so intensively as it does in us and in the animals, nevertheless, there too it becomes living oxygen. Oxygen under the earth is not the same as oxygen above the earth.

But we must now go farther. I have placed two things side by side; on the one hand there is the carbon structure which manifests the workings of the highest spiritual essence that is accessible to us on earth—the human ego, or the cosmic spiritual being which is at work in the plants. Observe the human process. We have breathing—living oxygen as it occurs inside the human being, living oxygen carrying the etheric. And in the background we have the carbon structure, which in the human being is in perpetual movement. These two must come together. The oxygen must somehow find its way along the paths mapped out by the structure.

The mediator is none other than nitrogen. Nitrogen guides life into the form or configuration that is embodied in the carbon.[49] Wherever nitrogen occurs, its task is to mediate between life and the spiritual essence which to begin with is in carbon. Everywhere—in the animal kingdom, in the plants and even in the earth—the bridge between carbon and oxygen is built by nitrogen. And the spirituality which—once again with the help of sulphur— is working thus in nitrogen is what we describe as the astral. It is the astral spirituality in the human astral body. It is the astral spirituality in the earth's environment. For as you know, there too the astral is working—in the life of plants and animals, and so on.

Thus, spiritually speaking, we have the astral placed between oxygen and carbon, and this astral impresses itself upon the physical by making use of nitrogen. Nitrogen enables it to work physically. The astral extends to wherever nitrogen is. The etheric principle of life would flow away everywhere like a cloud, it would take no account of the carbon structure were it not for nitrogen. Nitrogen has an immense power of attraction for the carbon structure. Wherever the lines are traced and the paths mapped out in carbon, there nitrogen carries the oxygen, there the astral in the nitrogen drags the etheric.

Nitrogen is for ever dragging the living to the spiritual

principle. That is why nitrogen is so essential to the life of the soul in the human being. For the soul itself is the mediator between the spirit and the mere principle of life.

Now you can see into the human breathing process. Through it the human being receives into himself oxygen — that is, the etheric life. Then comes the internal nitrogen and carries the oxygen everywhere where there is carbon, wherever there is something formed and figured, albeit in perpetual change and movement. That is where the nitrogen carries the oxygen, so that it can fetch the carbon and get rid of it. Nitrogen is the real mediator for the oxygen which is to be turned into carbon dioxide and breathed out.

At this point I think you will have a true idea of the necessity of nitrogen for the life of plants. The plant as it stands before us in the soil has only a physical and an etheric body; unlike the animal, it does not have an astral body within it. Nevertheless, outside it the astral must be there everywhere. The plant would never blossom if the astral did not touch it from outside. Though it does not absorb it (as the human being and the animals do), the plant must nevertheless be touched by the astral from outside. The astral is everywhere, and nitrogen itself — the bearer of the astral — is everywhere, moving about as a corpse in the air. But the moment it enters the earth, it is alive again. Just as with oxygen, so too nitrogen becomes alive; indeed, in the earth it grows in sentience and sensitiveness. Strange as it may sound, nitrogen not only becomes alive but sensitive inside the earth; and this is of the greatest importance for agriculture. Nitrogen becomes the bearer of that mysterious sensitiveness that flows over the whole life of the earth.

You have seen how there is living interaction. On the one hand there is what works out of the spirit in the carbon principle, taking on forms as of a scaffolding or structure. This is in constant interplay with what works out of the astral in the nitrogen principle, permeating the structure with inner life, making it sentient. And in all this, life itself is working through the oxygen principle. But these things can only work together in the earthly realm inasmuch as it is permeated by yet another principle, which for our physical world establishes the connection with the wide spaces of the cosmos.

There must be constant interchange of substance between the earth — with all its creatures — and the entire universe. All that is living in physical forms upon the earth must eventually be led back again into the great universe. It must be able to be purified and cleansed in the wide reaches of the cosmos.[50]

All that is thus developed in the living creature, structurally as in a fine and delicate design, must eventually be able to vanish again. It is not the spirit that vanishes, but that which the spirit has built into the carbon, drawing life to itself out of the oxygen as it does so. This must be able once more to disappear, not only in the sense that it vanishes on earth — it must be able to vanish into the cosmos.

We may describe the process thus. In all these structures, the spiritual has become physical. It lives in the body astrally, it lives in its image as the spirit or the ego — living in a physical way as spirit transmuted into the physical. After a time, however, it no longer feels comfortable there. It wants to dissolve again. And now once more — moistening itself with sulphur — it needs a substance in which it can abandon all structure and definition and find its way outwards into the undefined chaos or indistinguishable realms of the cosmos, where there is no organization of any kind.

This is achieved by a substance which is as nearly like the physical and yet again as nearly alike to the spiritual. The substance which is so near to the spiritual on the one hand and to the substantial on the other is hydrogen. Hydrogen carries out into the far spaces of the universe all that is formed and alive and astral. Hydrogen carries it upwards and outwards till it becomes such in nature that it can be received in the universe once more. It is hydrogen which dissolves everything away.[51]

6. Soil and the World of Spirit

George Adams once wrote 'the plant reveals the earth receiving and again resigning the formative influences of the spiritual universe in daily, yearly and other rhythms'. This chapter, examining the soil, the plant and its seed aims to offer a means by which such an imagination might be understood. We read firstly why a living quality within the soil is vital for its sensitivity to cosmic energies. This is of the greatest current relevance, for if soils become over-mineralized in character they will be increasingly 'deaf' to cosmic influences from the outer planets, leading to a one-sided, watery uptake of nutrient.

We hear of atmospheric nitrogen becoming 'living' within the soil, this being a metaphor of what happens to all substances when they are taken up by living organisms. Steiner stresses the importance of organic nitrogen in our fertilizers so it clearly is important to consider whether any substance has been connected previously with life processes or has a purely mineral or synthetic origin. Steiner talks about compost — not always by name — including compost-making and its benefit to plants either in terms of mineral substances or life forces. We also read of the intimate relationship of plant roots and soil, prefiguring much of what is now known about the nature and value of symbiotic soil micro-organisms such as mycorrhizae and bacterial nodules.

In so much of Steiner's work the influence of spiritual beings of the stars or planets of the cosmos is indicated; very little, by contrast, is mentioned about the apparent 'emptiness' of space. In the second part of this chapter we are challenged to visualize what cannot be seen but which surrounds and penetrates everything. This is surely no easier to comprehend than the nature of a supreme being. Steiner thus offers an explanation of what centuries ago was understood by the word 'chaos' and he points to its essential part in the creation of all new life and inspiration. It is of great importance in the penetration of matter by the spirit and we encounter this in the soil when the seed with its cosmic imprint needs to be influenced by counteracting forces from the earth. It is also to the chaos that all life returns when it is over.

Nurturing the life of the soil

The idea that in farming we are really exploiting the land is quite correct. Indeed, we cannot help doing so. With all that we send out into the world from our farms we are taking forces away from the earth – indeed, even from the air. These forces must somehow be restored.

No one realizes today that all the mineral fertilizers are precisely what contributes most to the degeneration of the products of agriculture. Nowadays people simply think that a certain amount of nitrogen is needed for plant growth, and they imagine it makes no difference how it's prepared or where it comes from.

People will discover that using inorganic fertilizers is

something that must eventually stop altogether. Any mineral fertilizer gradually reduces the nutritive value of whatever is grown on the fields where it is used; that is a general law. However, even the measures I have indicated,[52] if you now carry them out, will make it unnecessary to manure more than once every three years. Perhaps you will only need to do it every four to six years. You will be able to do without artificial fertilizers altogether, if only because they will become an unnecessary expense. Artificial fertilizer is something that will not be needed any more, so in time it will disappear.

Where fertilizer comes from, however, is not a matter of indifference. There is a big difference between the dead nitrogen that is found in the air along with oxygen, and another kind of nitrogen. I am sure you would not deny that there is a difference between a human corpse and a person who is alive and walking around — one of them is dead, the other is alive and ensouled. The same thing applies to nitrogen and to other substances. Dead nitrogen is mixed with the oxygen in the air around us and plays a role in our entire breathing process and interaction with the air. This kind of nitrogen cannot be alive for the simple reason that if it was, if we had to live in air that was alive, we would always be unconscious. In order for people to be conscious and think clearly, the air they breathe has to be dead; both its nitrogen and its oxygen have to be dead. But the nitrogen in the soil, the nitrogen that must enter the soil with the manure, this nitrogen must be formed under the influence of the entire heavens; this nitrogen must be alive. Thus there are two kinds of nitrogen: the nitrogen above ground, which is dead, and the nitrogen below ground, which is alive.[53]

Manuring and everything of the kind consists essentially of this, that a certain degree of life must be communicated to the soil, and yet more than life. In manuring, we must bring to the earth kingdom enough nitrogen to carry the life to those structures in the earth kingdom which need it — below the plant where the plant soil has to be.

There is one fact that can already give you a strong indication of what is needed. If you use purely mineral substances as manure, you will never get at the real earthly element; you will penetrate at most to the watery element of the earth. With mineral manures you can influence the watery content of the earth, but you do not penetrate sufficiently to bring to life the earth element itself. Plants, therefore, which have mineral manures applied will have the kind of growth that betrays the fact that it is supported only by a vitalized watery substance, not by a vitalized earthly substance.[54]

We can best approach these matters by beginning with the most basic kind of manure. I mean compost, which is sometimes even treated with scorn. In compost we have a means of kindling the life within the earth itself. We include in compost any kind of waste matter to which little value is attached; farm and garden refuse, grass that we have let decay, fallen leaves or the like, indeed even dead animals. These things preserve something not only of the etheric but even of the astral.[55] Living etheric and astral elements are contained in it—though not so intensely as in manure or in liquid manure, yet in a more stable form. The etheric and astral settle down more firmly in the compost, especially the astral.

In recent times, efforts have been made to investigate the working of bacteria—the smallest of living entities. We must regard these minute living entities as occurring by virtue of the processes that arise of themselves in the manure. The presence of these creatures may therefore be an extremely useful indication of the prevalence of such and such conditions in the manure itself. But there can be no great benefit in planting or breeding them. We should always remain in larger spheres for the life which is so vital to agriculture, and even to these minutest of creatures we should apply as little as possible of atomistic forms of thought.[56]

Now there is something, the excellence of which with regard to nature I have already described to you from several standpoints, and that is the chalky or limestone element. Bring some of this, perhaps in the form of lime, into the compost heap and you will get this result: without inducing too great evaporation of the astral, the etheric is absorbed by the lime and thus oxygen too is drawn in; the astral is made splendidly effective.[57]

You thereby obtain quite a specific result. When you manure the soil with this compost, you communicate to it something which tends very strongly to permeate the earthly element with the astral, without going by the roundabout way of the etheric. The astral, without first passing via the etheric, penetrates strongly into the earthly element.

Whenever in any given locality you have a general level separating what is above the earth from the interior, all that is raised above this normal level of the locality will show a special tendency to life — a tendency to permeate itself with etheric vitality. Hence you will find it easier to infuse ordinary inorganic mineral earth with fruitful humus or with any waste product in process of decomposition efficiently if you create mounds of earth, and infuse these with such substances. For then the earthy material itself will tend to become inwardly alive — like the plant.[58] The same process takes place in the growth of trees. The earth itself is 'hollowed upwards' to surround the plant with its etheric and living properties.

I am telling you this to familiarize you with the idea of the intimate connection between what is contained within the contours of the plant and what constitutes the soil around it. It is simply untrue that the plant's life ceases at its outer periphery. Its actual life is continued, especially from the roots of the plant, into the surrounding soil. For many plants there is no hard and fast line between the life within the plant and the life of the surrounding soil in which it lives.

We must thoroughly understand this idea if we want to understand the nature of manured earth or of earth treated in some similar way. To manure the earth is to make it alive, so that the plant will not be placed into dead earth and find it difficult out of its own vitality to achieve all that is necessary up to the fruiting process. The plant will more easily achieve what is necessary for the fruiting process if it is immersed from the outset in an element of life.[59] Fundamentally, all plant-growth has a slightly parasitic quality. It grows like a parasite out of the living earth. And it must be so.[60]

It has been considered beneficial in modern times to treat manure in various ways with inorganic substances — compounds or elements. So long as we try to improve the quality of manure by mineralizing methods we shall only succeed in vitalizing the liquid element — the water. For a sound plant structure it is necessary not only to vitalize the water — we must vitalize the earth directly, and this we cannot do by merely mineral procedures. We can only do this by working with organic matter, bringing it into such a condition that it is able to organize and vitalize the solid earthy element itself. To endow the mass of manure, or the liquid manure, with this kind of vitality or stimulus is precisely the object of those suggestions we are able to give to agriculture on the basis of spiritual science.[61] Such vitalization, such stimulation can be given to any material that is available as manure, provided we remain within the sphere of life.

There is a saying you will often find repeated in agricultural literature: 'Nitrogen, phosphoric acid, calcium, potash, chlorine, etc., even iron — all these are essential in the soil if plant growth is to prosper. Silicic acid, on the other hand, lead, arsenic, mercury' — and they even include soda in this category — 'at most have the value of stimulants or irritants for plant life.'

What is the truth in this connection? Great nature does not leave us in the lurch to such a great extent if we fail to take the silicic acid, lead, mercury or arsenic into account as she does if we fail to take into account potash, limestone or phosphoric acid. Heaven provides silicic acid, lead, mercury and arsenic — provides them freely with the rain. On the other hand, to have the proper phosphoric acid, potash and limestone content in the earth, we must till the soil and manure it properly.

Nevertheless, by prolonged tillage we can gradually impoverish the soil. We are, of course, constantly impoverishing it, and that is why we have to manure it. But the compensation through manuring may over time become inadequate — and this is happening today on many farms.[62] In such a situation we are ruthlessly exploiting the earth; we let it become permanently impoverished. We must then ensure that the true nature process can take place once more in the right way.

Those that are commonly called the stimulant effects are indeed the most important of all. Precisely the substances people think non-essential are present all around the earth — actively working, though in the finest dilution. Moreover, the plants need them just as much as they need what comes to them from the earth. They draw them in from the cosmic surroundings. Mercury, arsenic, silicic acid — these substances the plants suck upwards from the soil of the earth after they have been radiated into the soil from the cosmos.[63]

The resonance of chaos and cosmos

One important thing should be understood with regard to tilling the soil. We must comprehend the conditions under which the forces from cosmic spaces are able to pour down into the earthly realm. To recognize these, let us take our start from the seed-forming process. The seed out of which the embryo develops is usually regarded as a very complicated molecular structure; for after all, out of its complexity the whole new organism will grow. The new organism was already prefigured in the embryonic condition of the seed. Therefore this microscopic or ultra-microscopic substance must also be infinitely complex in its structure. This is true to a certain extent. When the earthly protein is built up, the molecular structure is indeed raised to the highest complexity. But a new organism could never arise out of this complexity. The organism does not arise out of the seed in that way. What develops as the seed out of the mother plant or mother animal does not simply continue its existence in what afterwards arises as the descendant plant or animal.

When the complexity of structure has been enhanced to the highest degree, it all disintegrates and eventually we have a tiny realm of chaos where we first had the highest complexity attained within the earth domain. It disintegrates, as we might say, into cosmic dust. When the seed — having been raised to the highest complexity — has fallen apart into cosmic dust and the tiny realm of chaos is there, then the entire surrounding universe begins to work and makes its imprint upon the seed, thus building up out of the tiny chaos what can only be built by forces flowing in from the great universe from all sides. In the seed we have an image of the universe.

In every seed formation the earthly process of organization is carried to the very end — to the point of chaos. Time and again the new organism is built up out of the whole universe in the chaos of the seed. The parent organism has this part to play — through its affinity to a particular cosmic situation, it brings the seed into a situation whereby the forces work from the right cosmic directions.

What is imaged in the single plant is always the image of some cosmic constellation. Ever and again it is built out of the cosmos. Therefore, if we want to make the forces of the cosmos effective in our earthly realm, we must drive the earthly as far as possible into a state of chaos. With regard to plant growth, nature will to some extent see that this is done. Since every new organism is built out of the cosmos, it is necessary for us to preserve the cosmic process in the organism until seed formation occurs.

Say we plant the seed of some plant in the soil. Here in this seed we have the stamp or impress of the cosmos from a given aspect. The constellation takes effect in the seed; thereby it receives its special form. The moment it is planted in the soil, the external forces of the earth influence it very strongly and it is permeated at every moment with a longing to deny the cosmic process.

When the first beginnings of the plant are unfolding out of the seed, and at later stages also, we need to bring the earthly element into the plant over against the cosmic form which is living as the plant form in the seed. We must bring the plant nearer to the earth in its growth. And this we can only do by bringing into the plant such life as is already present on the earth. That is to say, we must bring into it life that has not yet reached the chaotic state — life which came to an end in the organization of some plant *before* it reached the point of seed-formation.

In this respect a rich humus formation comes to our assistance. To what is humus formation due? It is due to the fact that the element which comes from plant life is absorbed by the whole process of nature. All life that has not yet reached the state of chaos to some extent rejects cosmic influences. The cosmic process works in the stream which passes upwards to the seed formation, while the earthly process works in the unfolding of leaf, blossom and so on — the cosmic only radiates its influence into all this. The reason why a leaf or grain absorbs inner substance lies in all that we bring to the plant by way of earthly life that has not yet reached the state of chaos. On the other hand, the seed which evolves its force right up the stem irradiates the leaf and blossom of the plant with the force of the cosmos.

Sulphur, carbon, nitrogen, hydrogen — all are united

together in protein. Wherever these occur—in leaf or flower, calyx or root—everywhere they are bound to other substances in one form or another. There are only two ways in which they can become independent: on the one hand, when hydrogen carries them outwards into the far spaces of the universe, separates them all, carries them all away and merges them into the universal chaos;[64] and on the other hand, when the hydrogen drives these fundamental substances of protein into the tiny seed formations and makes them independent there, so that they become receptive to the inflowing forces of the cosmos. In the tiny seed formations there is chaos and away in the far periphery there is chaos once more. Chaos in the seed must interact with chaos in the farthest periphery of the universe. Then the new being arises.

Chaos—a name borrowed from ancient times—really lies behind even what we understand as heaven. Not only the wonderful old Greek myth speaks of chaos when it says that the most ancient gods were born out of the chaos; the legends and myths of other nations too are acquainted with chaos.

All of us are familiar with a word which many people believe to be very old—the term 'gas'. Gas and 'gaseous' were unknown concepts before the time of the Rosicrucians Comenius and Helmont. It was in the case of carbon dioxide that Helmont first realized the nature of gas. Helmont came to the idea that among the states of substance there is also the gaseous state and in his work *Ortus Medicinale* (1615) we find the following sentence:

'This spirit which was hitherto unknown, I will name with a new name: Gas.' We can learn a great deal from this sentence. Helmont calls what he describes as gas *Spiritum* or spirit. That is to say, the transparent substance he has constituted is for him the instrument for a spiritual being.

Hence we can understand how much Helmont recognized in the process by which a gas is cooled and condensed. Miniature worlds arose from the gas for Helmont. In contemplating this world he said to himself: how did all this that is here originally come to be? Originally it arose from something that one cannot see, from out of which, however, as from a gas, the universe was formed. Once upon a time, the whole universe was *Spiritum*, purely spiritual. As the clouds of misty vapour are formed out of the gas, so out of the transparent, radiant, unclouded infinity of the spiritual all things that now exist emerged.

This ancient idea contains quite another concept of spirit than people have today. Space to them was not a great infinite void in which there is absolutely nothing; space was the all-spreading spirit whose parable they saw in the unclouded gas. In it they saw the source from which all seeds of things are created and spring forth through the Word of the original Divine Spirit.

Helmont coined the word 'gas' from the word 'chaos'. It is an extremely interesting connection in the world order. We are thus led by Helmont to a living conception of space, not empty and infertile like the concept of space for people today, but a concept of space appearing infinitely fertile bearing countless seeds. The infinitude that is spread out is the seed from which we issue. Everything that is in the world is space condensed; it is the infinite spirit who shows himself to us in place of mere empty space. Imagine how originally the pure, spiritual, transparent space was there. What happened in this pure transparent space? In this same space is also the extended gaseous air. As the thoughts that rise from our soul bring the air around us into vibration when they are spoken in the word, and every word shapes itself into forms in the air quite silently and unseen by us, so the Spirit of God hovered over the waters. Into the waters the creating words of the Godhead were spoken.

But the chaos is active not only in the beginning of world evolution; it works on and on; it is present even today. Just as around us are the harmonies of the spheres, the harmonious heavens, so all around us is the chaos, all things are permeated by it. It was the first and original foundation. Then it became cloudy; the seeds were formed; the shapes and forms arose; worlds were formed out of the chaos. But just as when a gaseous mass condenses something remains behind that works on between the single condensing particles, so likewise of the original spirit something remained behind. And so the chaos works on and lives on, along with the world. Everything is still permeated by the chaos—every stone, every plant, every animal is permeated by it. Our soul and our spirit are permeated with the chaos. The soul and the spirit of the human being also participate in the chaos.

This chaos is at the same time the essential reason for

the constant and ever-present fertility in nature. The working of chaos appears wherever animal excrement occurs. The new year's crop grows from the ploughed land after manure has been put into it—manure which lends the land fertility and causes the crop to grow and thrive. What has happened in such a case? What was the manure to begin with? The manure too was perhaps at one time a beautiful, marvellously formed plant, an entity in the world that had also once been formed out of the chaos. Then it served as nourishment for the animals and the useless substances were excreted again. Now the manure mingles with the soil; it is a return of beings into chaos. Chaos is working in manure, in all that is cast out; and unless at some time or other you mingle chaos with the cosmos, further evolution is never possible. The process we have before us here at its lowest level will enable us to rise to an understanding of the word 'chaos' with respect to higher realms. Cosmos cannot work alone. Everything in the cosmos has grown from causes, from things that went before—not only all physical things, but intellectual and moral teachings too arise from causes that were planted once before.[65]

It is cosmos when a Goethe, a Schiller, a Lessing have done their work. When a schoolmaster comes and assimilates and passes on all the beautiful things that are found in the works of these great men, he can only do so because the causes are already there for him. But with the human being of genius it is not so; he works out of the chaos. New impulses, new entries into evolution, new concepts arise and begin to take effect. Genius is like a fresh spark; it is out of the ordinary precisely because a union takes place there between the cosmos and the chaos; thereby a new thing arises not connected with the laws of evolution that come from ancient times. It enters from other worlds like a divine spark. Genius is the marriage of the past with the present, of the cosmos with the chaos.

We feel the overwhelming influence of the chaos that contains the seed of all things when we let these things work upon us. Thus we can see how comprehensive the idea of chaos is for anyone who understands it in the right way. It is chaos from out of which the physical arises. Be it Greek philosophy or the Bible, be it the Indian philosophy of the A-Chaos, the Akasha, all this reminds us that the element which was in the beginning works throughout all time.

7. Supporting and Regulating Life Processes

After laying the foundations, Steiner in his Agriculture Course *concerns himself with practical ways in which we can effect some degree of control in regard to nature's processes. He counsels us to build a living quality into our soil in order to make it more sensitive for the working of cosmic forces. He makes clear on other occasions that we shall reach a time when crop growing will become very difficult. Under these circumstances, methods to stimulate the flow of energies, as with acupuncture, will become more vital than at the present time. The first two suggestions are for vitalizing soil and root systems (horn manure preparation) and for the upward growth and ripening process of plants (horn silica). We are working here with polarities in the plant — the downward sensing within the root realm and the upward striving of stem, leaves and flower. In order to remain healthy, a plant must experience a balance in the operation of these principles which link respectively with the lime and silica principles introduced in Chapter 5. The remaining six preparations, of which four will be included here, enliven and balance the transformative processes taking place within compost and which afterwards continue their influence on the land. These compost preparations connect with particular planetary and nutrient processes and Steiner says that without a proper balance of planetary forces our protein will not be properly formed.*

We also learn how we can reduce the all-important lunar and planetary fertilizing influences in order to exercise control, in a non-chemical way, over problems which every farmer has with weeds and pests. Here we learn that just as water is fundamental to life, so fire can be made to bring about an opposing effect. We are made aware that when employing such methods their effectiveness is enhanced by observing the most auspicious cosmic times.

Field sprays to invigorate soil and plant

In dung we have before us something etheric and astral. For this reason it has a life-giving and also astralizing influence upon the soil, and, what is more, in the earth element itself — not only in the watery but notably in the earthly element. It has the force to overcome what is inorganic in the earthly element.[66]

We take manure such as we have available. We push it into the horn of a cow and bury the horn a certain depth into the earth. You see, by burying the horn with its filling of manure, we preserve in the horn the forces it was accustomed to exert within the cow itself, namely, the property of raying back whatever is life-giving and astral. Through the fact that it is outwardly surrounded by the earth, all the radiation that tends to etherealize and astralize is poured into the inner hollow of the horn. And the manure inside the horn is inwardly vitalized with these forces, which thus gather up and attract from the surrounding earth all that is etheric and life-giving.

And so, throughout the winter — in the season when the earth is most alive — the entire content of the horn becomes inwardly alive. All that is living is stored up in this manure. Thus in the content of the horn we get a highly concentrated, life-giving manuring force.

When it has spent the winter in the earth, you take the manure out of the horn and dilute it with ordinary water — only the water should perhaps be slightly warmed.

You must, however, thoroughly mix the entire content of the horn with water. That is to say, you must set to work and stir. Stir quickly, at the very edge of the pail, so that a crater is formed reaching very nearly to the bottom of the pail, and the entire contents are rapidly rotating. Then quickly reverse the direction, so that it now seethes round in the opposite direction.[67] Do this for an hour and you will get a thorough penetration.

Our next task will be to spray it over the tilled land so as to unite it with the earthly realm.[68]

The method I have just described can be followed up at once by another, namely, the following. Once more you take the horns of cows. This time, however, you fill them not with manure but with quartz or silica or even feldspar, ground to a fine mealy powder, say, of the consistency of a very thin dough. With this you fill the horn. And now, instead of letting it 'hibernate', you let the horn spend the summer in the earth and in the late autumn dig it out and keep its contents till the following spring.[69]

Then you dig out what has been exposed to the summery life within the earth, and you treat it in a similar way. Only in this case you need far smaller quantities. You can take a fragment the size of a pea, or maybe only the size of a pin's head, and distribute it by stirring it up well in a bucket of water. Here again, you will have to stir it for an hour, and you can now use it to sprinkle the plants externally. It will prove most beneficial with vegetables and the like.

Vitalizing solid or liquid organic fertilizers

We need to treat our manure[70] not only as I indicated on other occasions; we should also subject it to a further treatment. The point is not merely to add substances to it with the idea that it needs substances so as to give them to the plants. No, the point is that we should add living forces to it. The living forces are far more important for the plant than the mere substance forces or substances. Though we might gradually get our soil ever so rich in this or that substance, it would still be of no use for plant growth, unless by a proper manuring process we endowed the plant with the power to receive into its body the influences that the soil contains.

Today I shall mention a few more preparations to add to the manure in minute doses. These preparations vitalize it in such a way that it will be able to transmit its vitality to the soil from which the plants grow.

Take yarrow (*Achillea millefolium*), a plant that is

generally obtainable. It contains what the spirit always uses to moisten its fingers when it wants to carry the different substances to their several organic places. Yarrow stands out in nature as though some creator of the plant world had had it before him as a model, to show him how to bring sulphur into a correct relationship to the remaining substances of the plant.

Now you can do the following. Take the part of the yarrow that is medicinally used, namely, the upper part—the umbrella-shaped inflorescence. Take one or two handfuls, pressed strongly together, and sew it up in the bladder of a stag.[71] Now hang it up throughout the summer in a place exposed to the sunshine. When autumn comes, take it down again and bury it not very deep in the earth throughout the winter.

So you will have the yarrow flower enclosed in the bladder of the stag for a whole year, and exposed—partly above the earth, partly below—to those influences to which it is susceptible. You will find that it assumes a peculiar consistency during the winter.

In this form you can now keep it as long as you wish. Add the substance which you take out of the bladder to a pile of manure—it could even be as big as a house!—and distribute it well. Indeed, you need not even do much to distribute it—the radiation itself will do the work.[72]

The substance we thus gain from the yarrow has an effect so vitalizing and refreshing that if we now use the manure thus treated just in the way manure is ordinarily used we will make good again much that would otherwise become ruthless exploitation of the earth. We endow the manure with the power to vitalize the earth so that substances deriving from the more distant cosmos—silicic acid, lead, etc., which come to the earth in finest homoeopathic quantities—are caught up and received.

The bladder of the stag is connected with the forces of the cosmos. Indeed, it is almost an image of the cosmos. We thereby give the yarrow the power to enhance the forces it already possesses, to combine sulphur with the other substances.

Now take another example. We want to give the manure the power to receive so much life into itself that it is able to transmit life to the soil out of which the plant is growing. But we must also make the manure able to bind together to a greater extent the substances which are necessary for plant growth—that is, the calcium in addition to potash. If we also wish to get hold of calcium influences, we need another plant. This plant is camomile (*Matricaria recucita*). It is not enough to say that camomile is distinguished by its strong potash and calcium contents. The facts are these: yarrow mainly develops its sulphur force in the formative process associated with potash. Hence it has sulphur in the precise proportions that are necessary to assimilate the potash. Camomile, however, additionally assimilates calcium. Thereby it assimilates what can help exclude from the plant the harmful effects of fructification, thus keeping the plant in a healthy condition.

Now trace, for example, the process which camomile

undergoes in the human and animal organism when taken as food or medicine. The bladder is comparatively unimportant for what happens to camomile in the human or animal organism. In this case, the substance of the intestinal wall is far more important. Therefore, if you want to work with camomile you must proceed as follows.

Pick the beautiful delicate little yellow-white heads of the flowers and treat them as you treated the umbels of the yarrow. But now, instead of putting them in a bladder, stuff them into bovine intestines. You will not need very much. Instead of using these intestinal tubes as they are commonly used for making sausages, fill them with the stuffing which you thus prepare from the camomile flowers.

This preparation once again needs only to be correctly exposed to the influences of nature. Observe how we constantly remain within the living realm. In this case, living vitality connected as nearly as possible with earthly nature must be allowed to work upon the substance. Therefore you should take these precious little sausages and expose them to the earth throughout the winter.

Dig them out in the springtime and keep them in the same way as before. Add them to the manure just as you did the yarrow-preparation. You will thus get a manure with a more stable nitrogen content and with the added virtue of kindling the life in the earth, so that the earth itself will have a wonderfully stimulating effect on plant growth. Above all, you will create more healthy plants if you manure in this way than if you do not.

Most difficult to replace for its good influence on our manure is the stinging nettle. It is truly the greatest benefactor of plant growth. If it should happen to be unobtainable, then you must get it dried from elsewhere. The stinging nettle is a regular 'Jack-of-all-trades'. It can do very, very much. It, too, carries within it the element that incorporates the spiritual and assimilates it everywhere, namely, sulphur, the significance of which I have explained already. Moreover, the stinging nettle carries potassium and calcium in its currents and radiations, and in addition it has a kind of iron radiation. These iron radiations of the nettle are almost as beneficial to the whole course of nature as the iron radiations in our blood. The stinging nettle is truly a good fellow and does not deserve the contempt with which we often look down on it where it grows wild in nature. It should really grow around the human being's heart, for in the world outside — in its marvellous inner working and organization — it is wonderfully similar to what the heart is in the human organism. The stinging nettle is the greatest boon.

Now, to improve your manure still more, take any stinging nettles you can get, let them fade a little and press together slightly. Bury in the earth, adding a layer of peatmoss or the like, so as to protect it from direct contact with the soil. Bury it straight in the earth, but take good note of the place, so that when you afterwards dig it out again you will not be digging out mere soil. Let it spend the winter there and the following summer — it must be buried for a whole year.

This substance will now be extremely effective. Mix it with the manure, just as you did the other preparations. The general effect will be such that the manure becomes inwardly sensitive — truly sensitive and sentient, we might almost say intelligent. It will not suffer undue decomposition to take place within it — any inappropriate loss of nitrogen or the like.

The soil will individualize itself in relationship to the particular plants that you are growing. It is like infusing the soil with reason and intelligence, which you can bring about by such addition of *Urtica dioica*.

I know quite well that those who have studied academic agriculture from the modern point of view will say: 'You have still not told us how to improve the nitrogen content of the manure.' On the contrary, I have been speaking of it all the time, namely, in speaking of yarrow, camomile and stinging nettle. For there is a hidden alchemy in the organic process. This hidden alchemy really transmutes the potash, for example, into nitrogen, provided only that the potash is working properly in the organic process. Indeed, it even transforms limestone, the chalky nature, into nitrogen if it is working properly.

You know that all the four elements of which I have been speaking are involved in the growth of plants. Hydrogen is also there, in addition to sulphur. I have told you of the significance of hydrogen. Now there is a mutual and qualitative relationship between limestone and hydrogen, similar to that between oxygen and nitrogen in the air.

Even externally, in a quantitative chemical analysis, the relationship between the oxygen-nitrogen connection in the air and the limestone-hydrogen connection in the organic processes could be revealed. The fact is that, under the influence of hydrogen, limestone and potash are constantly being transmuted into something very like nitrogen, and at length into actual nitrogen.[73] And the nitrogen that is formed in this way is of the greatest benefit to plant growth. We must enable it to be thus engendered by methods such as I have here described.

Silicon, too, is transmuted in the living organism — transmuted into a substance of great importance, which, however, is not yet included among the chemical elements at all. We need the silicic acid[74] to attract and draw in the cosmic properties. Now in the plant there simply must arise a clear and visible interaction between the silicic acid and the potassium — not the calcium. By the whole way in which we manure the soil we must vitalize it so that the soil itself will aid in this relationship.[75]

We must now look for a plant which by its own relationship to potassium and silicic acid can impart to the manure a corresponding power. This, too, is a plant which, even if it only grows wild on our farms, has a most beneficial influence in this direction. It is none other than the dandelion (*Taraxacum officinale*).

This dandelion is truly a kind of messenger of heaven. But if we want to make it effective in the manure we must use it in the right way. Gather the little yellow heads of the dandelion, press them together, sew them up in a bovine mesentery and let them lie in the earth throughout the winter. In springtime you take the balls out and can keep them until you need them. They are now thoroughly saturated with cosmic influences. The substance you get out of them can once again be added to the manure. It will give the soil the ability to attract as much silicic acid from the atmosphere and the cosmos as the plants need to make them really sentient. They of themselves will then attract what they need.

To be able to grow truly, plants must have a kind of sensitivity. Even as I, a human being, can pass by a dull person and he will not notice me, so too all that is in the soil and above it will pass a dull plant by; and the plant will fail to sense it, will not, therefore, enlist it in the service of its growth. But if the plant is finely permeated and vitalized with silicic acid, it will grow sensitive to all things, and will draw to itself all that it needs.

Treat the soil as I have now described, and the plant will draw things to itself from a wide circle. Your plant will then benefit not only from what is in the field in which it grows, but also from that which is in the soil of the adjacent meadow or neighbouring wood or forest. That is what happens once it has thus become inwardly sensitive. We can bring about a wonderful interplay in nature by giving plants the forces that come to them through the dandelion in this way.

Suppressing the growth of weeds

We shall get the strongest of weeds if we let the kind moon work down upon them and do nothing to arrest its influence. For there are wet years when the moon forces work more than in the dry. The weeds will then reproduce themselves and increase greatly.

If, on the other hand, we reckon with these cosmic forces we can contrive to check the full influence of the moon upon the weeds. We must only let work upon them the influences coming from without—not the moon influences, but those that work directly. Then we shall set a limit to the propagation of the weeds; they will be unable to reproduce themselves. Now we cannot 'switch off' the moon. Therefore we must treat the soil in such a way that the earth is disinclined to receive the lunar influences. Indeed, not only the earth but the plants too can become disinclined to receive the lunar influences. We can make the weeds reluctant, in a sense, to grow in soil that has thus been treated.

You see the weeds growing rampant in a given year. You must accept the fact. Do not be alarmed; say to yourself: something must now be done. So now you gather a number of seeds of the weed in question. For in the seed the force of which I have just spoken has reached its final culmination. Now light a flame—a simple wood-flame is best—and burn the seeds. Carefully gather all the resulting ash. You get comparatively little ash, but that does not matter. Quite literally, by letting seeds pass through fire and turn to ash you will have concentrated the opposite forces to those of the moon.

Now use the tiny amount of substance you have thus prepared from a variety of weeds, and scatter it over your fields. You need not take special care in doing so, for these things work in a wide circumference.[76] As early as in the second year you will see that there is far less of the weed you have treated. It no longer grows as rampantly. Moreover, many things in nature being subject to a cycle of four years, after the fourth year you will see, if you continue sprinkling the preparation year by year, the weed will have ceased to exist on the field in question. Here you are producing a result based on the 'effect of smallest entities', which has now been scientifically proven in our Biological Institute.[77]

Generally speaking, you have far-reaching possibilities if you take these influences into account. People today will not believe these things; such things were known and mastered once upon a time by an instinctive farming wisdom. They could plant together, in defined areas, whatever they wanted to have. They knew of these things instinctively. In all these matters, I can only give indications but these indications are capable of direct practical application.

Just as water on the one hand is a *sine qua non* of all fertility, so fire on the other hand is an absolute destroyer of fertility. Fire consumes fertility. Therefore, if you treat by fire in the proper way that which is normally treated by water to bring about fertility in the plant-world, you will bring about destruction. A seed will develop fertility in large scope through moon-saturated water; likewise, a seed will develop forces of annihilation in large scope through moon-saturated fire—and in general through cosmically saturated fire.

After all, the fact that we count upon this great force of dispersal (while pointing out the precise effects of time in the process) need not seem utterly strange to you. The force of the seed always works in dispersal and expansion. Hence it works far and wide in the force of annihilation too. Expansive power lies inherently in the nature of the seed. It is the very property of the seed to have this power of dispersal; so, too, the preparation we make in this way has a real expansive power.

Regulating the abundance of pests

We are able to speak in general terms of the harmful plant or vegetable pests of the field. But we can no longer speak so generally when we come to animal pests. Let me choose one example, the field mouse.

It is not quite sufficient to apply what we need to do in such a case to a single farm by itself, though to some extent it may help even then. It will not be very easy to carry out. One has to try and come to an agreement so that one's neighbours will do it as well. You catch a fairly young mouse and skin it, so as to get the skin. But you must obtain this skin of the field mouse at a time when Venus is in the sign of Scorpio.

The people of olden times, you see, were not so stupid with their instinctive science! Now that we are passing from plants to animals, we come to the 'animal circle' — that is, the zodiac. It was called so not without reason. To achieve our purpose within the plant world we can stop at the planetary system. For the animal world, that is not enough. There we need ideas that take the surrounding sphere of the fixed stars, notably, the fixed stars of the zodiac, into account.

Moreover, in the growth of plants the moon influence is more or less sufficient to bring about the reproductive process. In the animal kingdom, on the other hand, the moon influence must be supported by that of Venus. Indeed, for the animal kingdom the moon influence does not need to be considered very much. For the animal kingdom conserves the lunar forces; it emancipates itself from the moon. The moon force is developed in the animal kingdom even when it does not happen to be full moon. The animal carries the force of the full moon within it, conserves it, and so emancipates itself from limitations of time.

This does not apply to what needs to be done here; it does not apply to the other planetary forces. For you must do something quite definite with the mouse skin. At the time when Venus is in Scorpio, you obtain the skin of the mouse and burn it. Carefully collect the ash and the other constituents that remain over from the burning. It will not be much, but if you have a number of mice it will be enough.

Thus you obtain your burned mouse skin at the time when Venus is in Scorpio. And there remains in what is thus destroyed by the fire the corresponding negative force as against the reproductive power of the field mouse. Take the preparation you get in this way, and sprinkle it over your fields. In some districts it may be difficult to carry out; then you can afford to do it even more homoeopathically; you do not need a whole plateful.

Provided it has been led through the fire at the high conjunction of Venus and Scorpio[78] you will find this an excellent remedy. Henceforth, your mice will avoid the field. No doubt they are cheeky little beasts; they will soon come out again if the preparation has been so sprinkled that a few areas remain unsprinkled in the neighbourhood. There they will settle down again. The influence of the preparation does undoubtedly ray out; nevertheless, it may not have been done thoroughly. The effect will certainly be radical if the method is applied to the whole neighbourhood.

Mice are rodents; they are included among the higher animals. But you will not achieve much with insects in this way. Insects are subject to different cosmic influences. In such a case you do not take part of the insect as you do with the mouse. You must take the entire insect. It is best to burn it; that is the quickest way. You might also let it decay; possibly this would be even more thorough, only it is difficult to collect the products of decay. But you will certainly attain what you need by burning the whole insect.

Now it is necessary to perform this operation when the Sun is in the sign of Taurus. (If need be, you can keep the insect and burn it when the time comes.) This, you see, is precisely the opposite of the constellation in which Venus must be when you prepare your mouse skin preparation. The insect world is connected with the forces that evolve when the sun is passing through Aquarius, Pisces, Aries, Gemini, and on to Cancer. In Cancer the effect is quite weak, and it is weak again when you come to Aquarius. It is while passing through these regions that the sun rays out the forces that relate to the insect world.

8. Spirits of the Elements

In previous chapters reference has been made to cosmic forces or energies that have seemed fairly inanimate. But when Rudolf Steiner spoke of such life-formative energies – otherwise known as etheric formative forces or astral forces – he did not intend us to think only of abstract forces and their effects. We might search for scientific evidence of their existence and come to equate such forces with cosmic rays, the wavelength of which is 10 million times shorter than visible light. However, the ultimate reality is that these fine energies arise from the impulses of higher beings and are mediated by nature spirits or elemental beings. These spirits therefore become the intermediaries between the creative will of beings of the hierarchies and the unfolding of life on earth. They help to explain why processes take place rather than simply how.

As will be apparent from what follows, these beings completely sacrifice themselves in the cause of supporting life and providing nourishment for beings of the physical world. We may think of them as being enchanted by the diverse forms they help create. Steiner says that in their entirety they constitute the etheric body of the earth and that the human etheric body is also connected with a range of such beings. We shall see that the elemental spirits are those which fully experience the earth's breathing rhythms.

When we look at the plant, each of the primal life elements comes to expression in the different organs, roots, leaves, flowers and seeds. Each of these has an elemental being directing its activities. Finally, we discover that not only are these beings responsible for bringing new life into existence but they have ways of offering up their labours to enable the hierarchies to experience something of the creative work they have carried out.

Elementals as the manifestations of cosmic forces

An earlier, instinctive vision beheld the beings of the supersensible world as well as those in the world of the senses. Today, these beings have withdrawn from human view. The reason why this company of gnomes, undines, sylphs and fire spirits[79] is not perceptible in the same way as animals, plants, and so on, is merely that the human being, in the present epoch of Earth evolution, is not in a position to unfold his soul and spirit without the help of his physical and ether bodies. In the present situation, the human being is obliged to depend on the etheric body for the purposes of his soul, and on the physical body for the purposes of his spirit. The physical body, which provides the instrument for the spirit, that is, the sensory apparatus, is not able to enter into communication with the beings that exist behind the physical world. It is the same with the etheric body, which the human being needs to develop as an ensouled being. As a consequence, half of his earthly environment escapes him. He passes over everything connected with elemental beings. The physical and the ether body have no access to this world.[80]

Easter occurs at the time of the bursting and sprouting life of spring. At this time the earth is breathing out its soul forces in order that these soul forces may be permeated again by the astral element surrounding the earth, the extra-earthly, cosmic element. The earth is breathing out its soul. What does this mean?

It means that certain elemental beings, which are just as much in the periphery of the earth as the air is, or as the forces of growth are—that these unite their own being with the exhaled earth soul in those regions in which it is spring. These beings float and merge with the exhaled earth soul. They lose their individuality and rise in the general earthly soul element.

During Easter time we see them come together in a general cloud and form a common mass within the earth soul. But by so doing these elemental beings lose their consciousness to a certain degree and enter into a sort of sleeping condition. Certain animals sleep in the winter; these elemental beings sleep in summer. This sleep is deepest during St John's time, when they are completely asleep. Then they begin once more to individualize, and when the earth breathes in again at Michaelmas, at the end of September, we can see them already as separate beings again.[81]

The human being needs these elemental beings. This is not in his consciousness, but the human being needs them nonetheless in order to unite them with himself so that he can prepare his future. And the human being could unite these elemental beings with himself if at a certain festival time—it would have to be at the end of September—he could perceive with a special inner liveliness how nature herself changes towards the autumn, if he could perceive how the animal and plant life recedes, how certain animals begin to seek their shelters against the winter, how the plant leaves get their autumn colouring, how all nature fades and withers.

As soon as we ascend into the ether, we encounter warmth ether, light ether, chemical ether and life ether. If we look at these kinds of ether with the spiritual vision that sees elemental beings, we find the elemental beings of the etheric spheres. We find light beings. We find number beings, and we find the beings who let life stream through the cosmos and who carry it. These beings are quite different from the beings in the lower elemental kingdoms. We should point to the fact that just as the lower elements—earth, water, air and warmth—are populated by elemental beings, so there are other beings in the etheric elements: light ether, chemical ether and life ether.[82]

Spiritual beings, who can also be called elemental beings, are enchanted in the air and are bewitched into a lower form of existence when air is transformed into the liquid state. An enchantment of spiritual beings is always connected with the condensation and formation of gases and solids. How can divine spiritual beings create solid, liquid and airy substances as they exist on our planet?

They send down elemental beings; they imprison them in air, water and earth. These are the elemental messengers of the spiritual, creative, formative beings. These beings to whom we owe everything surrounding us are enchanted in the objects we see.

The nature spirits, the descendants of the beings of the third hierarchy, are master builders and foremen in the kingdoms of nature. Such elemental beings are messengers for the divine spiritual beings. They are involved in everything that occurs in the outer, perceptible world. What the elemental beings have called into the world is the last reverberation of the creative, formative, cosmic Word, which underlies all activity and all existence.[83]

Elemental beings of the plant kingdom

To the outwardly perceptible, visible world there belongs the invisible world, and the two of them, taken together, form a whole. The marked degree to which this is the case first appears in its full clarity when we turn our attention away from the animals to the plants.

Plant life, as it sprouts and springs forth from the earth, immediately arouses our delight, but it also provides access to something which we must feel to be full of mystery. In the case of the animal, though certainly its will and whole inner activity have something of the mysterious, we nevertheless recognize that this will is actually there and is the cause of the animal's form and outer characteristics. But in the case of the plants, some other factor must be present in order that this plant world may arise.

When spiritual vision is directed to the plant world, we are immediately led to a whole host of beings which were known and recognized in the old times of instinctive clairvoyance but which were afterwards forgotten and today remain only as names used by poets, names to which the modern human being ascribes no reality.[84] To the same degree, however, in which we deny reality to the beings that flit so busily around the plants, to that degree do we lose understanding of the plant world. This understanding of the plant world, which, for instance, would be so necessary for the practice of medicine, has been entirely lost.

Plants send down their roots into the ground. Anyone who can observe what they really send down, and can perceive the roots with spiritual vision, sees how the root is everywhere surrounded by the activities of elemental nature spirits. And these elemental spirits, which an old clairvoyant perception designated as gnomes and which we may call the root spirits, can actually be studied through Imagination and Inspiration,[85] just as human life and animal life can be studied in the physical world.

These root spirits, which are everywhere present in the earth, get a quite particular sense of well-being from rocks and from ores. They have the greatest feeling of well-being in this sphere because it is the place where they belong, where they are conveying what is mineral to the roots of the plants. And they are filled with an inner spirituality that we can only compare to the spirituality of the human eye and the human ear. They are entirely sense, and it is a sense which is at the same time intellect, which does not only see and hear but immediately understands.

We can even indicate the way in which these root spirits receive their ideas. We see a plant sprouting out of the earth. The plant enters into connection with the extra-terrestrial universe; and, particularly at certain seasons of the year, spiritual currents flow from the flower and the fruit of the plant down into the root, streaming into the earth. And just as we turn our eyes towards the light and see, so do the root spirits turn their faculty of perception towards what trickles downwards from above through the plant into the earth. What trickles down towards the root spirits is something which the light has sent into the flowers, which the heat of the sun has sent into the plants, which the air has produced in the leaves, which the distant stars have brought about in creating the plant form. The plant gathers the secrets of the universe, sends them into the ground, and the gnomes take these secrets into themselves. And because the gnomes, particularly from autumn and through the winter, in their wanderings through ore and rock, bear within them what has trickled down through the plants, they are the bearers of the ideas of the universe, of the cosmos, inside the earth. But they have no liking at all for the earth itself. They flit about in the earth with cosmic ideas, but they actually dislike what is earthly.

The gnomes are really the element within the earth that represents the extra-terrestrial, because they must continually avoid growing together with the earthly. And it is from this feeling of hatred, of antipathy towards the earthly, that the gnomes gain the power of driving the plants up from the earth. The antipathy causes the plant to have only its roots in the earth and to grow out of the earth; in fact, the gnomes force the plants out of their true, original form and make them grow upwards and out of the earth.

Once the plant has grown upwards, once it has left the domain of the gnomes and has passed out of the sphere of the element of moist earth into the sphere of moist air, the plant develops what comes to outer physical form in the leaves. Other beings are at work in everything that goes on in the leaves — water spirits, elemental spirits of the watery element, to which an earlier clairvoyance gave, among others, the name of undines. Just as we found gnome beings flitting busily around the roots, we see close to the soil these water beings who observe with pleasure the upward-striving growth that the gnomes have produced.

These undines differ in their inner nature from the gnomes. They cannot turn outwards towards the universe like a spiritual sense organ. They can only yield themselves up to the movement and activity of the whole cosmos in the element of air and moisture and they therefore do not have the clarity of mind that the gnomes have. They dream incessantly but their dream is at the same time their own form.

In dreaming their own existence they bind and release, they bind and separate the substances of the air, which in a mysterious way they introduce into the leaves. They take these substances to the plants that the gnomes have thrust upwards. The plants would wither at this point if it were not for the undines, who approach from all sides, and as they move around the plants in their dreamlike consciousness they prove to be what we can only call world chemists.

To the same degree, however, in which the plant grows into the dream of the undines, it now enters into another domain higher up, into the domain of the spirits that live in the element of air and warmth. In the element of air and warmth live the beings that an earlier clairvoyant faculty called the sylphs. Because air is everywhere imbued with light, these sylphs living in the element of air and warmth press towards the light and become related to it. They are particularly susceptible to movements within the atmosphere. The sylphs, which experience existence more or less in a state of sleep, feel most in their element, most at home, where birds are winging through the air.

The sylph feels its ego through what the bird sets in motion as it flies through the air. Because its ego is kindled in it from outside, the sylph becomes the bearer of cosmic love through the atmosphere. Thus we behold the deepest sympathy between the sylphs and the bird world. The gnome hates the amphibian world—the undine is sensitive to fishes. The sylph, on the other hand, is attracted towards birds and has a sense of well-being when it can waft towards their feathered flight the floating air filled with sound.

Through the fact that the sylphs bear light into the plant, something quite remarkable is brought about. The sylph is continually carrying light into the plant. The light, that is to say the power of the sylphs in the plant, works on the chemical forces that were induced in the plant by the undines. Here the interaction of the sylph's light and the undine's chemistry occurs. This is a remarkable moulding and shaping activity. With the help of the substances streaming up that are worked on by the undines, the sylphs weave an ideal plant form out of the light.

After it has passed through the sphere of the sylphs, the plant enters the sphere of fire spirits. These inhabit the element of heat and light. When the warmth of the earth is at its height, or has reached a sufficient level, it is gathered up by the fire spirits. Just as the sylphs gather up the light, so do the fire spirits gather up the warmth and carry it into the flowers of the plant.

Undines carry the action of chemical ether into the plants, sylphs the action of light ether into the flowers. And the pollen provides what may be called little airships that enable the fire spirits to carry warmth into the seed. Everywhere warmth is collected with the help of the stamens, and is carried by means of the pollen from the anthers to the seeds in the carpel.

For plants the earth is the mother, the heavens the father. And all that takes place outside the domain of the earth is not the maternal womb for the plant. It is a colossal error to believe that the maternal principle of the plant is in the carpel. This is in fact the male principle which has been drawn forth from the universe with the aid of the fire spirits. The maternal element is taken from the cambium of the plant, which lies between bark and wood.

Because people do not recognize what is spiritual, do not know that gnomes, undines, sylphs and fire spirits are actively involved in plant growth, there is a complete lack of clarity about the process of fertilization in the plant world. With the help of what comes from the fire spirits, the gnomes down below instil life into the plant and push it upwards. They are the fosterers of life. They carry the life ether to the root—the same life ether in which they themselves live. The undines foster the chemical ether in the plant, the sylphs the light ether, the fire spirits the warmth ether. And then the fruit of the warmth ether again unites with what is present below as life. Thus plants can only be understood when they are considered in connection with all that is flitting around them full of life and activity.

In order to carry the concentrated warmth, which must descend into the earth so that it may be united with the plant's ideal form, the fire spirits feel themselves intimately related to the butterfly world, and to the world of the insects in general. Everywhere they follow in the tracks of the insects as they flit from flower to flower.[86] When a bee flies through the air from plant to plant, from tree to tree, it flies with an aura that is actually given to it by a fire spirit.

This, you see, is the spiritual process of plant growth.

And it is because the subconscious in the human being divines something of a special nature in the flowering, sprouting plant that he experiences the being of the plant as full of mystery.[87]

We now see that the earth is indebted for its power of repulse and impulse regarding growth as well as its density to the antipathies of the gnomes and undines.[88] If the earth is dense, this density is due to the antipathy by means of which the gnomes and undines maintain their form. When light and warmth come down to earth, this is at the same time an expression of that power of sympathy, that sustaining power of sylph love, which is carried through the air, and to the sustaining sacrificial power of the fire spirits, which brings the power to descend to what is below. So we may say that over the earth's face, earth density, earth magnetism and earth gravity in their upwardly striving aspect unite with the downward striving power of love and sacrifice. And in this interaction of the downward streaming force of love and sacrifice and the upward streaming force of density, gravity and magnetism, in this interaction where the two streams meet, plant life develops on the surface of the earth. Plant life is an outer expression of the interaction of world love, world sacrifice, world gravity and world magnetism.

Elementals as gatherers of substance

The ancestors of our earth gnomes, the moon gnomes, gathered together their moon experiences and from them fashioned the solid structure of the earth. The gnomes acquire an extraordinarily interesting relationship to the whole evolution of the universe. They preserve the solid structure from one cosmic body to another. It is one of the most interesting studies to examine these supersensible, spiritual beings and to observe their special task, for this gives one a first impression of how every kind of being shares in the task of working on the whole form and structure of the world.

Let us pass to the undines. These beings do not have the need for life that human beings have but one could almost say that the undines, and also the sylphs, only feel themselves to be truly alive when they die.

We see the remarkable fact that each year, with the return of early spring, these beings evolve upwards from unfathomable depths. There they take part in the life of the earth by working on the plant kingdom. Then however they take up by means of their own bodily nature the phosphorescence of the water, the decaying matter, and bear it upwards with an intensity of longing. Then, in a magnificent cosmic picture, one sees how — emanating from earthly water — the colours carried upwards by the undines with spiritual substantiality provide the higher hierarchies with their sustenance, how the earth becomes a source of nourishment in that the very essence of the undines' longing is to let themselves be consumed by higher beings.[89]

And now let us proceed to the sylphs. In the course of the year birds die. I described to you how dying birds possess spiritualized substance, and how they desire to give this spiritualized substance over to higher worlds in order to release it from the earth. But here an intermediary is needed. And these intermediaries are the sylphs. It is a fact that dying birds continually fill the air with astrality.

And when we go on to the fire spirits, just think how the dust on the butterfly's wings seems to dissolve into nothing with the death of the butterfly. But it does not really dissolve into nothing. What is shed as dust from the butterfly's wings is the most highly spiritualized matter. And all this passes like microscopic comets into the warmth ether that surrounds the earth. When in the course of the year the butterfly world approaches its end, all this becomes an inner glittering and shimmering. And the fire spirits pour themselves into this glittering and shimmering; they absorb it. There it continues to glitter and shimmer, and they too get a feeling of longing. They bear what they have thus absorbed up into the heights. And now one sees — I have already described this to you from another aspect — how the glittering and shimmering carried outwards from the butterfly's wings by the fire spirits shines forth into cosmic space. But it does not only shine forth; it streams forth. And it is this which provides the particular view of the earth which the higher hierarchies perceive. The beings of the higher hierarchies gaze upon the earth, and what they principally see is this butterfly and insect existence which has been carried outwards by the fire spirits; and the fire spirits find their highest bliss in the realization that it is they who present themselves before the spiritual eyes of the higher hierarchies. They find their highest bliss in being beheld by the gaze, by the spiritual eyes, of the higher hierarchies, in being absorbed into them. They strive upwards towards these beings and carry to them knowledge of the earth.

Thus we see how these elemental beings are the intermediaries between the earth and the spirit cosmos.[90]

9. Nutrition and Vitality

A fundamental point of divergence between Steiner's picture of nutrition and the orthodox one is his distinction between earthly and cosmic nutrition streams applying to animals and human beings. Hence what is eaten has only an indirect relationship to what happens in the body. To a large extent we require food as a fuel to give the bodily processes the capacity to carry out their tasks — to provide immediate or slower-released energy for example — while bodily substance results mainly from the absorption of cosmic ethers through our system of sense organs.

Earthly food actually has a threefold function: it provides energy, it provides the physical substance of the brain and nerve system, and it provides what can be likened to a blueprint in the etheric body for the renewal of the body's substance by way of the cosmic stream. This connects especially with protein formation and raises the issue of why the quality of our food is of such importance. This quality or vitality affects the body's capacity to engage vigorously with the repair and re-formation of substances out of the cosmos and to build a strong auto-immune system, which we associate with good health. It is with food produced according to principles already discussed that the body is granted these forces in the appropriate way. Interaction thus occurs between the two forms of nutrition in all of the body's metabolic processes and in this respect the human etheric body, astral body and ego participate in different aspects of this overall process.[91]

We first present a brief cameo of these new concepts, aiming also to connect with themes of earlier chapters. The main elements of our diet and how they relate to the processes of digestion are then examined in more detail. We will note the ease with which minerals can be taken into the body — as dissolved salts — whereas carbohydrates, fats and proteins require progressively greater breakdown in order to be utilized. We also learn that there is a nutritional relationship — albeit of a generalized kind — between the separate parts of plants and different sections of our bodies. This constitutes a further step towards a healthier nutrition and towards treating a certain range of illnesses.

Finally, these various principles are applied to the nutrition and care of animals. This is essential knowledge following a lengthy period of intensification of animal production. Specialized breeding has clearly deserved greater attention to nutrition than it has received, while stressful living conditions are widespread and are a common cause of disease as well as reducing the quality of products for human consumption.

New concepts in nutrition

People believe that the most important part of nutrition is the food one eats, but the greatest part of what one eats every day is not there in order to be taken into the body as a substance; the greatest part is there in order to give the body the forces which one finds in it, and to bring the body into movement. On the other hand, what the body needs in order to provide itself with substances which are deposited in the body and which one expels again every seven or eight years as the bodily substances are renewed — the greatest part of this is taken in through the sense organs, through the skin, and through breathing. The substances the body has to take in and deposit in itself are constantly being absorbed in extremely small doses, which only become condensed inside the organism.[92] The body takes these from the air and hardens and condenses them, so that they then have to be cut off in one's nails and hair and so forth. It is wrong to think in terms of the formula: food taken in, passage through the body, flaking off of skin and nails and the like. The correct formulation is: breathing, absorption of the finest substances through the sense organs — including the eyes — passage through the organism, excretion. The importance of what we take in through the stomach lies in its inner mobility, like that of a fuel — for it brings will forces into the body which work in it.

Just as we have light, colour and sound sensations when we open our eyes or prick up our ears, so we are continually receiving impressions from the elemental world which produce imaginations in our etheric body. Even though these imaginations do not directly enter our consciousness in everyday life, they are more important for our whole life than sense perceptions, for we are much more intensely and intimately connected with our imaginations than with our sense perceptions. We belong to this elemental world, we receive our own etheric body from it, and the latter is an instrument for intercourse with this elemental world.

Our eyes are closely connected with the earth's light ether forces (sylphs), the sense of taste is connected with chemical ether forces (undines) and our sense of smell is connected with the earth's life ether (gnomes). The sense of warmth is connected with the warmth ether which radiates through space (fire spirits).[93]

Just as the etheric body is mainly situated in the abdomen and the astral body in the chest, so the ego is mainly situated in the head. We also have to see it like this: the physical body has to do with solid matter, the etheric body with the fluid, the astral body with the gaseous, and the ego with warmth.[94] Anything to do with the human being's ego brings warmth into motion. This can be traced in detail in the human body. The ego is also connected with the blood, and that is why the blood produces warmth.

The plant and the digestive process

A plant consists of root, leaf, stem, blossom and fruit. Now look at the root for a moment. It is in the earth. It contains many minerals and the root clings to the earth with its fine rootlets, so it is constantly absorbing those minerals. The root of the plant has a special relation to the mineral realm of earth.

The part of the human being that is related to the whole earth is the head—not the feet, but actually the head. When the human being starts to be on earth in the womb, he has at first almost nothing but head. His head takes the shape of the whole cosmos and the shape of the earth. The head particularly needs minerals. It is from the head that the forces go out that fill the human body with bones. You can see from this that we need roots. They are related to the soil and contain minerals. We need minerals for bone building. Bones consist of calcium carbonate, calcium phosphate; those are minerals. The human being needs roots in order to strengthen his head.

And so, if a child becomes weak in his head for instance — inattentive, hyperactive — he will usually have a corresponding symptom: worms in his intestines. Worms develop easily in the intestines if the head forces are too weak, because the head does not then work down strongly enough into the rest of the body.

Carrots are the root of the plant. They grow down in the earth and have a large quantity of minerals. They have the forces of the earth in them, and when they are taken into the stomach they are able to work up through the blood into the head. Only substances rich in minerals are able to reach the head. It is through carrots that the uppermost parts of the head become strong, which is precisely what the human being needs in order to be inwardly firm and vigorous.

When we eat a potato, we are really eating a piece of swollen, enlarged stem. The potato is something between the root and the stem. It does not have as much mineral content as the carrot; it is not as earthy. It contains carbohydrates in particular. When we eat potatoes, first they go into the mouth and stomach. There the body has to exert strength to derive starch from them. Then the digestive process goes further in the intestines. In order that something can go into the blood and also reach the head, there must be more exertion still, because sugar has to be derived from the starch. Only then can it go to the head. So one has to use still greater forces. Now think of this: when I exert my strength upon some external thing, I become weak. But if I exert an inner strength, transforming carbohydrates into starch and starch into sugar, I become strong. Precisely through the fact that I permeate myself with sugar by eating potatoes, I become strong. When I use my strength externally, I become weak; if I use it internally, I become strong. So it is not a matter of simply filling oneself up with food, but of the food generating strength in our body.

While the potato is a rather poor foodstuff, the grains — wheat, rye, and so on — are good foodstuffs. The grains also contain carbohydrates, and of such a nature that the human being forms starch and sugar in the healthiest possible way. Actually, the carbohydrates of the grains can make us stronger than we can make ourselves by any other means.

And now, what happens when we cook the grain? Well, when we cook the grain, we eat it warm. And it is a fact that to digest our food we need inner warmth. Unless there is warmth we cannot transform our carbohydrates into starch and the starch into sugar — that requires inner heat.

So if we first apply external heat to the foodstuffs, we help the body — it does not have to provide all the warmth itself. By being cooked, foods have already begun the warmth process. Think what happens to the grain when I make flour into bread. First I have ground the seeds. I have crushed them into tiny pieces. And what I do there with the seeds, grinding them, I would otherwise have to do later within my own body. Everything I do externally, I would otherwise have to do internally; so by doing those things, I relieve my body. And the same applies to all the things I do in cooking. I bring the foods to a condition in which my body can more easily digest them.

But now, let us come to the fats. Plants, almost all of them, contain fats. Fats do not enter the human body so easily as carbohydrates and minerals. When fats are eaten, they are almost entirely transformed by the saliva, by gastric and intestinal secretions, and they become something quite different that then goes over into the blood. Animal and human beings must form their own fats with forces which the fats they eat call forth. With the fats that he eats, the human being develops strength by destroying the substances.

But now let us think how it is when someone eats the stems and leaves of a plant. When he eats green matter, he is getting fats from the plants. And the greener that leaves are, the more fats they have in them. So when someone eats bread, for instance, he cannot take in many fats. He takes in more, for example, from watercress. That is how the custom came about of putting butter on our bread, some kind of fat. It was not just for the taste.

That, I would say, is the secret of human nutrition: that if I want to work upon my head, I have roots or stems for dinner. If I want to work upon my heart or my lungs, I make myself a green salad. And in this case, because these substances are destroyed in the intestines and only their forces proceed to work, cooking is not so necessary. That is why leaves can be eaten raw as salad. Lettuce and similar things work particularly on heart and lungs, building them up, nourishing them through the fats.[95] Whatever is to work on the head cannot be eaten raw; it must be cooked. Cooked foods work particularly on the head.[96]

But the human being must not only nurture the head and the middle body, or chest region, he must nurture the digestive organs themselves. He needs a stomach, intestines, kidneys and a liver, and he must build up these digestive organs himself. Now the interesting fact is this: to build up his digestive organs he needs protein, the protein that is in plants, particularly as contained in their blossoms and especially in their fruit. So we can say: the root nourishes the head particularly; the middle of the plant—stem and leaves—nourishes the chest particularly; and fruit nourishes the lower body.

Cast an eye up at the plums and apples, at the fruits growing on the trees—those we do not have to bother to cook much, for they have been cooked by the sun itself. There, an inner ripening has already been happening, so that they are something quite different from the roots or from stalks and stems, which are not ripened but actually dried up by the sun. The fruits we do not have to cook much—unless we have a weak organism, in which case the intestines cannot destroy the fruits.

You can see what a good instinct human beings have had for these things. Naturally they have not known in concepts all that I have been telling you—they have known it instinctively. They have always prepared a mixed diet of roots, greens and fruit; they have eaten all of them, and even the comparative amounts that one should have of these three different foods have been properly determined.[97] But now, as you know, people not only eat plants, they eat animals too, the flesh of animals, animal fat and so on. Most people are really unable to produce their own fat if they have only plant fats to destroy. Plant fats do not go out beyond the intestines; they are destroyed in the intestines. But the fat contained in meat does go beyond, it goes over into the human being. And the person may be weaker than if he were on a diet of just plant fats.

There are people who simply cannot live if they do not have meat. A person must consider carefully whether he really will be able to get on without it. If he does decide he can do without it and changes over from a meat to a vegetarian diet, he will feel stronger than he was before. That is sometimes a difficulty; obviously some people cannot bear the thought of living without meat. If, however, a person does become a vegetarian, he feels stronger because he is no longer obliged to deposit alien fat in his body; he makes his own fat, and this makes him feel stronger.

I know this from my own experience. I could not otherwise have endured the strenuous exertion of these last 24 years! I never could have travelled entire nights, for instance, and then given a lecture the next morning. For it is a fact that if one is a vegetarian one carries out a certain activity within one that is spared the non-vegetarian, who has it done first by an animal. That is the important difference.[98]

But I would never agitate for vegetarianism! It must always be first established whether a person is able to become a vegetarian or not; it is an individual matter.

When I eat roots, their minerals go up into my head. When I eat salad greens, their forces go to my chest, lungs, and heart—not their fats, but the forces from their fats. When I eat fruit, the protein from the fruit stays in the intestines. And the protein from animal substances goes beyond the intestines into the body; animal protein spreads out. One might think, therefore, that if a person eats plenty of protein, he will be a well-nourished individual. This led to the fact in this materialistic age that people who had studied medicine were recommending excessive amounts of protein for the average diet.

If one gulps down too much protein, it does not go over into the body at all, but into the faecal waste matter. Before it passes out, it lies there in the intestines and poisons the whole body. That is what can happen from too much protein. And from this poisoning, arteriosclerosis very frequently results—so that many people get arteriosclerosis too early simply from stuffing themselves with too much protein.

The point is really that one must know how the various substances work. One must know that minerals work particularly on the head; carbohydrates—just as they are to be found in our most common foods, bread and potatoes, for instance—work more on the lung and throat system (lungs, throat, palate and so on). Fats work particularly on heart and blood vessels, arteries and veins, and protein particularly on the abdominal organs.

A human being takes salt into his body and it travels all the way to his head in such a way that the salt remains salt. It is really not changed except that it is dissolved. It keeps its forces as salt all the way to the human head. In contrast to this, protein—the protein in ordinary hens' eggs, for instance, but also the protein from plants—this protein is at once broken down in the human body while it is still in the stomach and intestines; it does not remain protein. The human being possesses forces by which he is able to break down this protein. He also has the forces to build something up again, to make his own protein. He would not be able to do this if he had not already broken down other protein.

Now think how it is with such protein. Imagine that you have become exceptionally clever, so clever that you can make a watch. But you have never seen a watch except from the outside, so you cannot immediately make a watch. But if you take it all apart and lay out the pieces in such a way that you observe how the parts relate to one another, then you know how to put them all together again. That is what the human body does with protein. It must take in protein and take it all apart.

Protein consists of carbon, nitrogen, oxygen, hydrogen and sulphur. Those are its most important components. And now the protein is completely separated into its parts, so that when it all reaches the intestines, the human being does not have protein in him, but he has carbon, nitrogen, oxygen, hydrogen and sulphur.

One must always be eating new protein in order to be able to make protein. The fact is, the human being is involved in a very, very complicated activity when he manufactures his own protein. First he divides the protein he has eaten into its separate parts and puts the carbon from it into his body everywhere. Now you already know that we inhale oxygen from the air and that this oxygen combines with the carbon we have in us from proteins and other food elements. And we exhale carbon in carbon dioxide, keeping a part of it back. So now we have that carbon and oxygen together in our body. We do not retain and use the oxygen that was in the protein; we use the oxygen we have inhaled to combine with the carbon. Thus we do not make our own protein as the materialists describe it.

Again, we do not use the nitrogen that comes to us in the hens' eggs; we use the nitrogen we breathe in from the air. And we do not use the hydrogen we have eaten in eggs. We use the hydrogen we take in through our nose and our ears, through all our senses; that is the hydrogen we use to make our protein. Sulphur too — we receive that continually from the air. Hydrogen and sulphur we get from the air. From the protein we eat, we keep and use only the carbon. There is a similar situation with fat. For the fats too, we use very little nitrogen from our food.

We must take care to bring healthy plant protein into our body. Healthy plant protein! If a person wants to keep himself healthy, it is really necessary to include fruit in his diet. If he neglects to eat fruit, he will gradually condemn his body to a very sluggish digestion.

It is also a question of giving proper nourishment to the plants themselves. And that means we must realize that plants are living things; they are not minerals, they are something alive. A plant comes to us out of the seed we put in the ground. The plant cannot flourish unless the soil itself is to some degree alive. And how do we make the soil alive? By manuring it properly. Yes, proper manuring is what will give us really good plant protein.[99]

The nutrition and health of animals

The significance of nutrition for the animal, and for the human being too, is to this day thoroughly misunderstood. The coarse idea that the foodstuffs are received from outside and then deposited in the organism is altogether wrong. That is what people imagine nowadays to a greater or lesser extent. True, they conceive all kinds of transformations in the process, and yet, fundamentally speaking, that is how they think. The animal absorbs the food, deposits inside itself whatever it can use and excretes what it has no use for. Accordingly, we must provide for such and such essential constituents. We must see to it that the creature is not overburdened. We must see to it that the food it gets is as nutritive as possible, so that it can use a relatively large proportion of what it contains. True, people also distinguish between nutritive substances in the narrower sense and those which assist the combustion process in the body.

In the animal there is no such sharply outlined threefold structure of the organism as there is in the human being. True, in the animal the nervous and sensory organism and the metabolic and limb organism are well marked and sharply divided one from the other. But the middle, rhythmic organism more or less melts away — at least it does so in many animals. Something that still comes from the sensory organism passes into the rhythmic, likewise something that comes from the metabolic organism.[100]

Now all the substances that are present in the organization of the head are composed of earthly matter. On the other hand, all that we have as substance in the organization of the metabolism and the limbs — permeating our intestines, limbs, muscles, bones, and so forth — does not come from the earth at all. It is cosmic substance. It comes from that which is absorbed out of the air and warmth above the earth.[101] You must not regard a claw or a hoof as though it were formed by the physical matter which the animal eats somehow finding its way into the hoof and being deposited there. What the animal eats is merely for the purpose of developing its inner forces of movement, so that the cosmic principles may be driven right down into the metabolic and limb system.

Precisely the opposite is true of the forces. In the head we have cosmic forces because the senses are chiefly stationed there and the senses perceive out of the cosmos, while in the metabolic and limb systems we are dealing with earthly forces — cosmic substances and earthly forces. (As to the latter, you need only remember how we walk; we are constantly placing ourselves into the field of earthly gravity, and in like manner all that we do with our limbs is bound up with the earth.)

This is by no means a matter of indifference in practice. Suppose you are using an ox as a working animal — it is important to feed the animal so that it gets as much as possible of cosmic substance. Moreover, the food which will pass through the stomach must be suitably chosen so as to develop plentiful forces — forces sufficient to guide the cosmic substance into the limbs and bones and muscles, everywhere.

Likewise we need to be aware that whatever substances are required for the head must be acquired from the actual fodder. The foodstuffs — passed through the stomach — must be guided into the head. Moreover, the head can only assimilate this nourishment from the body if it is able to get the necessary forces from the cosmos. Therefore we should not merely shut our animals in dark stables where the cosmic forces cannot flow towards them. We should put them in pastures. Altogether, we should give them the opportunity to enter into a relationship with the surrounding world by sense perception too.

Think of an animal standing in a dark, dull stable and receiving measured out into its manger what the wisdom of the human being provides. How different will such an animal be from one that is able to make use of its senses, its organ of smell for instance: seeking its food for itself in the open air, following the cosmic forces through its sense of smell, going after the food, choosing for itself, unfolding all its activity in finding and taking its food.[102]

Such things are inherited. The animal you merely place at the manger will not reveal at once that it has no cosmic forces; for it still inherits them. But it will eventually produce descendants that no longer have the cosmic forces in them. In such a case it is from the head that the animal first becomes weak. It can no longer feed the body because it is unable to absorb the cosmic substances that, once again, are needed in the body as a whole.

We can now find the specific relationship of the animal organism to the plant. Observe the root, which develops inside the earth. There the manure permeates it with a nascent ego force—an ego force in process of developing. The root is assisted in absorbing this ego force if it can find the proper quantity of salt in the soil. On the basis of the thoughts we have already discussed, we can now recognize the root as that food which, if it enters the human organism, will most easily find its way to the head in the digestive process.

We will therefore provide root nourishment for the head so that the cosmic forces working plastically through the head may find the proper material to work upon. What does the following sentence remind you of: 'I must give roots as fodder to an animal that needs to carry material substance into its head, so that it may have a live and mobile relationship between its senses and the cosmic environment.' Do you not immediately think of the calf and the carrot? When the calf eats the carrot, this process is fulfilled.

Now that the material substance has been conveyed into the head, the reverse process must be able to take place. The head must be able to work with the will, creating forces in the organism, so that these forces in their turn can work right down into the body. The carrot dung must not be merely deposited in the head. From what is deposited there — from what is there in a process of disintegration — forces must radiate into the body. Therefore you need a second food.

Suppose, then, I have given carrot fodder. I want the body to be properly permeated by the forces that are able to evolve out of the head. I need something that has a raylike, radiating form, or that gathers up the raylike nature. So my attention is directed to linseed or the like. Such is the fodder you should give young cattle. Carrots and linseed, or something that will go together on the same principle, for instance carrots and fresh hay. These

will work through the animal, mastering its inner processes, setting it well on the way of its development.

Thus for young cattle we should always try to provide
fodder that will stimulate the ego forces on the one hand,
and on the other hand assist what passes downwards
from above — the astral radiations which are needed to fill
the body throughout. Assistance of the latter kind is provided especially by whatever is long and thin-stalked and
goes to hay.[103]

Let us pursue the matter further. Suppose you wish the
animal to become strong in the middle region. What
animals do you wish to become strong in this region? The
milk-giving creatures — they must grow strong in this
middle part.

What must you ensure in this case? You must see that
the right interaction exists between the stream that passes
backwards from the head, which is mainly a streaming of
forces, and the stream that passes forward from behind,
which is mainly a streaming of substance. If this interaction takes place such that the streaming from behind is
thoroughly worked through by the forces that flow from
the fore parts backwards, good and copious milk will be
the outcome.

For good milk production we must look to green
foliage. If we want to stimulate the development of milk in
an animal we will certainly attain the desired result if we
use plants that draw the fruiting process down into the
foliage. This applies to the pod-bearing or leguminous
plants, notably the various kinds of clover. Treat the cow

in this way and you will not see much result in the cow herself, but when she calves (for the changes in fodder you introduce along these lines generally take a generation to work themselves out), the calf will become a good dairy cow.

There is a wonderful instinct in these matters. Why did it ever occur to human beings to cook their food? Because they discovered that a considerable part is played in all that tends towards the fruiting process by such processes as cooking, burning, heating, drying, steaming. These processes will incline the flower, the seed and upper parts of the plant to develop more strongly the forces that have to be developed in the metabolic and limb systems of the animal. They work there chiefly by virtue of the forces they unfold, not by their substance. For the metabolic and limb systems require earthly forces, and to the extent that they need them they must receive them.

Think of the animals that pasture on the alpine meadows, for example. They are not like the animals of the plains, for they must walk about under difficult conditions. The conditions are different, simply through the fact that the earth's surface is not level. It is a different thing for animals to walk about on level ground or on a slope. Such animals, therefore, must receive what will develop the forces in the region of their limbs, i.e., the forces that have to be exerted by the will. Otherwise they will not become good work animals, or dairy or fattening animals.[104]

We must see to it that they get sufficient nourishment from the aromatic alpine herbs, where through the cooking process of the sun, working towards the flowers, nature herself has enhanced the fruiting, flowering activity by further treatment. But the necessary force can also be brought into the limbs by artificial treatment, notably through cooking, boiling, simmering or the like.

Now let us come to the question, how should we fatten animals? Here as much as possible of cosmic substance must be placed, as it were, into a sack. Oh, those pigs, those fat pigs and sows — what heavenly creatures they are! In their fat body — in so far as it is not the nervous and sensory system — they have nothing but cosmic substance. The pigs only need the material food they eat to distribute throughout their body this infinite fullness of cosmic substance which they must absorb from all quarters. The pig must feed so as to be able to distribute the substance which it draws in from the cosmos. It must have the necessary forces for the distribution of this cosmic substance.

And so it is with other fattened animals. Your fatstock will thrive if you give them fruiting substance — further treated, if possible, by cooking, steaming or the like.

This condition is on the whole fulfilled in certain oil-cakes and the like. But we must not leave the head of an animal unprovided for. Some earthly substance must be able to pass upwards into the head. We therefore additionally need something else, albeit in smaller quantities. We should therefore add something of a rooty nature (turnips or beet for instance) to the food of our fattening animals.

You can only proceed rationally by taking your start from a way of thought such as I have indicated, for this will very largely simplify the animal's food, and you will gain a comprehensive view of what you are doing. Think how you will approach your farming work if you do things in this way, quite consciously and deliberately. You will gain knowledge that does not complicate but simplifies the fodder problem.

Over the past few years, we have done many experiments with a medication used to treat foot-and-mouth disease in cattle.[105] These experiments were conducted on large farms as well as small ones, where the milk production for each cow was lower. You could find out all sorts of things because you had to try out the medication.

When you do these experiments, you will discover the following. Calves born to cows that are forced to produce too much milk are considerably weaker. You can observe this in the effect the medication has on the calf. The effectiveness or lack of effectiveness is greatly magnified. Eventually the calf grows up, if it does not die of disease. But a calf whose mother has been overfed in order to force it to give more milk is a much weaker calf than one whose mother was not forced to produce as much milk. You can observe this in the first, second, third and fourth generations. Then the calf gets to be so small that you hardly notice it. This type of forced milk production has not been in existence for very long, but I know one thing for certain, if people continue along this path, if a single cow is made to deliver over 30 litres of milk a day, if they continue to mistreat these animals this way, then after some time dairy farming may come to a bitter end. There is nothing that can be done about that.

Consider a cow or an ox. The ox itself has produced the flesh in its body from plant substances. This is the most important point to consider. This animal's body is therefore capable of producing meat from plants. Flesh is produced in the animal's body, and forces to do this must first be present in the body. With all our technological forces, we have none by which we can simply produce meat from plants. We do not have that, but in our bodies and in animal bodies there are forces that can make meat substance from plant substance.

Now, think of a plant that is still in a meadow or field. The forces that have been active up to this point have brought forth green leaves, berries, and so forth. Imagine a cow eats this plant. When the cow eats this plant, it becomes flesh in her. This means that the cow possesses the forces that can make this plant into meat.

Now imagine that an ox suddenly decided that it was too tiresome to graze and nibble plants, that it would let another animal eat them and do the work for it, and then it would eat the animal. In other words, the ox would begin to eat meat, though it could produce the meat by itself. It has the inner forces to do so. What would happen if the ox were to eat meat directly instead of plants? It would leave all the forces unused that produce the flesh in him. Think of the tremendous amount of energy that is lost when the machines in a factory in which something or other is manufactured are all turned on without producing anything. There is a tremendous loss of energy. But the unused energy in the ox's body cannot simply be lost, so the ox is finally filled with it, and this pent-up force does something in him other than produce flesh from plant substances. It does something else in him. After all, the energy remains; it is present in the animal, and so it produces waste products. Instead of flesh, harmful substances are produced. Therefore if an ox were suddenly to turn into a meat eater, it would fill itself with all kinds of harmful substances such as uric acid and urates. Now urates have their specific effects. The specific effects of urates are expressed in a particular affinity for the nervous system and the brain. The result is that if an ox were to consume meat directly, large amounts of urates would be secreted; they would enter the brain and the ox would go crazy. If an experiment could be made in which a herd of oxen were suddenly fed with pigeons, it would produce a completely mad herd of oxen. That is what would happen. In spite of the gentleness of the pigeons, the oxen would go mad.

The oxen would turn into terribly wild, furious creatures. This is proved by the fact that horses become extremely violent when fed a little meat. They begin to grow wild, because they are not accustomed to eating it.[106]

10. Responsibility for the Future

Steiner's spiritual science or anthroposophy gives us insight into future tasks which humankind must accomplish, tasks which to an extent depend on gaining the right nutrition. A major responsibility attaches to caring for the earth to enable it to provide a basis for our onward path. This places the knowledge offered to us through biodynamic agriculture at an important crossroads to our future. This chapter attempts to deepen the explanation of why a new direction in agriculture is so important and how it can be connected with progress in human development.

Those in a variety of movements are already committed to the task of saving the earth, and this feeling of responsibility among humanity is spreading. To such human energies must be added the deepened knowledge that can come from spiritual science. Indeed, Steiner makes clear that the earth and humanity are one, so besides the damage we do to the earth arising from our material existence we must realize that our moral outlook too has its repercussions on earth processes such as those of the crust and atmosphere.

The challenge for human beings is therefore to take responsibility for an inner development which comes about both by meditation and through our standards in daily life. In this way we consciously confront adversary forces and gain strength through developing hidden qualities. We then fulfil the needs of spiritual beings as well as developing closer attachment to elementals connected with nature's processes, thus reinforcing our efforts to care for outer nature.

Without understanding of this kind there can be little hope of progress towards longer-term goals. In the far future the human race must transform itself and spiritualize the earth. This aim might seem an area of potential dispute, raising as it does the issue of human freedom. Yet real freedom is misunderstood, and has more to do with the limitations we create for ourselves than the apparent strictures of a pre-determined plan. Each major phase in evolution has had a principal objective. It was towards the development of individual responsibility that the Buddha gave his great teachings. The task before us now according to Steiner is to fully develop the faculty of love, towards which the Christ-being, now united with the earth, offers a divine evolutionary impulse.

The inner challenge for human beings

In every human being there slumber faculties by means of which he can acquire for himself a knowledge of higher worlds. The mystic, the Gnostic, the theosophist,[107] have always spoken of a world of soul and a world of spirit which are as real to them as the world we see and touch. Anyone who listens to them may say to himself: I too can know if I develop certain powers which today still slumber within me.[108] It can only be a matter of how to set to work to develop such faculties. As long as a human race has existed, there has always been training, in the course of which individuals possessed of the higher faculties gave guidance to those who were seeking for them.

If we do not develop within ourselves the deeply rooted feeling that there is something higher than ourselves, we shall never find the strength to evolve to a higher stage. The heights of the spirit can be scaled only by passing through the gateway of humility. You can acquire true knowledge only when you have learnt to respect it.

Whoever has within him feelings of true devotion brings a great deal with him when he seeks access to higher knowledge. Our civilization tends more to criticism, judgement, condemnation than to devotion and selfless veneration. But every criticism, every adverse judgement passed, dispels the powers of the soul for the attainment of higher knowledge. This is not meant to imply anything against our civilization. To this critical faculty, this principle of 'prove all things and hold fast what is best' we owe the greatness of our culture. The human being could never have developed the science, industry, commerce and civil rights of our time if he had not everywhere exercised his critical faculty. But what we have gained in the way of external culture we have had to pay for with a corresponding forfeiture of higher knowledge, of spiritual life.

The treading of the path of knowledge by the pupil takes place silently, unnoticed by the outer world. He performs his duties and attends to his business as before. The transformation proceeds entirely in the inner recesses of the soul, hidden from outer sight. At first the pupil's whole inner life is filled by this basic mood of reverence for everything that is truly venerable. His whole life of soul finds its centre in this one basic feeling.

The pupil is advised to arrange moments in his daily life for withdrawing into himself, in stillness and alone. But during these moments he should not occupy himself with the affairs of his own ego — that would bring about the opposite of the aim in view. He should allow what he has experienced and what the outer world has said to him to echo in the stillness. Every flower, every animal, every action will then unveil to him secrets undreamed of. And thus he will begin to see the outer world with quite different eyes.[109]

The pupil does not learn in order to accumulate learning as his own treasure of knowledge, but in order to place this learning in the service of the world. Knowledge you pursue merely for the enrichment of your own learning and to accumulate treasure of your own leads you away from your path; but knowledge you pursue in order to grow more mature on the path of human ennoblement and world progress brings you a step forward.

No one is an authentic pupil of higher knowledge until he has made this the guideline of his whole life. This truth of spiritual training can be summed up in a short sentence: every idea that does not become your ideal kills a power in your soul; every idea that becomes an ideal engenders life forces within you.

Human influence on nature's processes

Things that take place through human influence, though they cannot be outwardly explained, are inwardly quite clear and transparent. Such things will come about as a result of practising meditation.[110] When you meditate you live quite differently with the nitrogen which contains the imaginations. You put yourself in a position which will enable these things to be effective with regard to the whole world of plant growth.

However, these things are no longer as clear today as they used to be in olden times, when they were universally accepted. For there were times when people knew that by certain definite practices they could make themselves fitted to tend the growth of plants. Nowadays, when such things are not observed, the presence of other people disturbs them. These delicate and subtle influences are lost when you are constantly living and moving among men and women who take no notice of such things. Hence, if you try to apply them, it is very easy to prove them fallacious.

A question was raised, namely, whether parasites could be combated by such means — by means of concentration or the like. You can, provided you do it in the right way. You would want to choose the proper season — from mid-January to mid-February — when the earth unfolds the forces that are most concentrated. Establish a kind of festival time, and practise certain concentrations during the season, and the effects might well be evident.

The only condition is that it must be done in harmony with nature as a whole. You should be well aware that it makes all the difference whether you do an exercise of concentration in the winter-time or at midsummer.[111]

A further task for human beings is to live consciously with the rhythm of the seasons, to experience nature in spring through the physical body, in summer through the etheric body, in autumn through the astral body, and in winter through the ego.[112]

Natural science provides a knowledge of the earthly that is confined to the connection between external causes and effects; and in this cycle of causes and effects, the human being too is involved. The fact that moral impulses also light up in the human being is admitted but nothing is known about the connection between these impulses and what comes to pass in external nature.

According to modern preconceptions there is something inexorable[113] in the play of nature, indeed pleasantly inexorable for materialistic thinkers. They imagine that the earth's course would be exactly the same were no human beings in existence, that whether they behave decently or not makes no difference. But that is not the case. The essential causes of what happens on the earth do not lie outside the human being; they lie within humankind. And if earthly consciousness is to expand to cosmic consciousness, humanity must realize that the earth is made over long stretches of time, in the likeness of humanity itself. There is no better means of lulling the human being to sleep than to impress upon him that he has no share in the course taken by earth existence.

If we observe the earth's crust and its vegetation correctly, we can see in the crystals, the mountains, the budding and sprouting plants monuments of a living, creative past which is now in process of dying. But in the human being we see the physical and etheric organism permeated with an astral body and ego throwing light across into the future and able to unfold freely a life of thought. In the human being we see past and future side by side. That element which already functions as future is the element that confers freedom; this freedom is not to be found in external nature.

If therefore nature is not to perish, she must be given what the human being has through the astral body and ego. This means that in order to ensure a future for the earth, human beings must insert into it the supersensible and invisible that we have within ourselves. Only when we place into the earth what it does not have itself, only then can an earth of the future arise. What is not there of itself is principally the active thoughts of human beings as they live and weave in our own organism. If we bring these thoughts to a real existence, we confer a future on the earth — but we must first have them. Thoughts that we have about ordinary nature are more reflections than realities. But thoughts guided from spiritual knowledge become forms that have an independent existence in the life of the earth.

Recognizing the needs of spiritual beings

The beings of the elemental kingdom—the gnomes, undines, sylphs, salamanders—help build up and form the plants. These beings were led and influenced by certain higher beings who are now withdrawing from this activity, just as at certain times these higher beings withdraw their influence within human beings and apply themselves to higher tasks. The elemental spirits are thus left to themselves, and other spirits (Lucifer, Ahriman) seize them and draw them away from their work in forming the plants. The result will be a diminution of the spiritual forces of the plants and a gradual atrophy, against which even artificial fertilizers will not help.

What must now be striven for is that human beings familiarize themselves with the elemental kingdom, that they attempt to establish a connection with these elemental spirits. In a sense, human beings must take over and prevent other powers from using the elemental kingdom and must strive to influence these spirits in such a way that they continue to assist in the growth of plants.[114] If human beings are able to cultivate these kinds of forces in themselves, they will become priests as farmers. If it is not possible to bring about such a connection, then in a few decades human beings will have to experience that the yield and quality of the products of the fields are diminishing and that no remedy can be found.[115]

The undines take part in the formation of dew. These

spirits too are on the verge of being drawn away from their previous activities by other beings. In time this would have the consequence that the formation of dew would gradually cease. Here too, human beings must strive to bring their influence to bear.

In order to gain a spiritual relationship to the animal kingdom, the human being must penetrate to the group souls of the animal genera. One can already perceive — and this will increase significantly — that the instincts of the animals are becoming weaker. For example, animals will no longer avoid poisonous plants in their fodder, but will rather eat them along with the rest. When human beings penetrate to the group souls, they can then compensate for the weakening of the animals' instincts; by this means the animals can be helped.

Now let us look at the world that surrounds us. The solid stones, the streams, the evaporating water that rises as mist, the air — all things that are solid, liquid or gaseous — are, in fact, densified fire. Gold, silver and copper are densified fire. In the far distant past everything was fire; everything was born of fire, but in all forms of densification spiritual beings lie enchanted.[116]

How are the divine beings that surround us able to produce solid matter as it exists on our planet? How do they produce liquid and airy substances? They send down elemental beings that dwell in fire and imprison them in the air, water and earth. They are emissaries, elemental messengers of the spiritual, creative beings.

Are human beings able to help these elemental beings in

some way or other? That is the great question that was put by the Holy Rishis. Are we able to release them? Yes, we can. For the deeds of the human being on earth are nothing but the external expression of spiritual processes. Everything we do here is also of importance for the spiritual world.

Something is continually passing from these elementals into the human being, and it goes on from morning until night. As we look out into the world, hosts of elementals who were or who are continually being enchanted into the processes of densification are continually entering into us from our surroundings.

Now let us assume that a person as he stares at an object has not the slightest inclination to reflect about what he sees or to let the spirit of things live in his soul. He does not digest his experiences spiritually by means of thoughts and feelings. In that case, elemental beings enter into him and remain there. They have gained nothing in the world process and have merely transferred their seat from the outer world into that of the human being. But now let us take a person who digests his impressions spiritually by thinking about them, and by forming concepts about the underlying spiritual foundation of the world. As a result of his spiritual activity he redeems the elemental being that streams towards him. He releases the elemental being from its enchantment. So through our spiritual activity we can release beings who are bewitched in air, water and earth and lead them back to their former condition, or we can imprison them in our inner being without any transformation having taken place in them. Throughout the whole of the human being's life on earth, elemental beings stream into him. It depends on him whether they remain unchanged or whether he releases them.

You meet someone and experience that he uses his perception, thinking — and what is in him of weaving, flowing thoughts enters his nervous system and is reflected in all perceptions, in sounds and colours. What, then, happens to this spirit light which enters into him? Here, we find the Cherubim gathering up this light to use in the service of the cosmic order — we are all light givers, forming part of the cosmic order. We are torchbearers of the spiritual world for the Cherubim; when we think, mental light radiates from us and illuminates the world in which the Cherubim live.

Everything we do is due to the fact that impulses of will work in us. What human activity does in the external world prompted by moral impulses is gathered up by the Seraphim. Such moral action is the source of warmth for the whole cosmic order. Under the influence of people whose actions are immoral the Seraphim freeze; that is to say, they do not receive the warmth needed to heat the whole cosmic world. Under the influence of moral action the Seraphim obtain forces by which the cosmic world order is maintained, just as the physical world is maintained through physical warmth.

You can see how the world conception provided by spiritual science becomes very real. We follow our path through the world, conscious that we do so not as useless good-for-nothings but having our place for the good of the whole cosmic order, while on the other hand we are at liberty to be a source of darkness in the world. For if we choose not to think, we increase the darkness; if we are immoral we increase the cold in the whole cosmic order.

Spiritual science does not just give us theories such as external science can do, unless it is practical science rightly applied. Spiritual science gives us something which teaches us to understand our true relationship to the whole cosmic order. Then something of vital importance results — it is a heightened sense of responsibility as regards the meaning of human existence.

The long-term goal of humanity

In the course of evolution, the whole of humanity will become capable of everything that the individual can achieve through occult training. But what will be happening to the earth while humankind is developing? There is a great difference between the earth seen by the esotericist and the earth known to the scientist. The latter regards it as a great lifeless ball with an interior not very unlike its exterior, except that the interior substances are fluid.[117] But it is not easy to understand how such a lifeless ball could have produced all the different kinds of beings on it. We know that on this earth of ours various phenomena occur which deeply affect the fate of many people. The fate of thousands may be affected by an earthquake or volcano. Does the human will have any influence on this, or is it all a matter of chance? Are there laws which act with blind fury, or is there some connection between these events and the will of the human being? What does the esotericist say about the interior of the earth?

We must think of the earth as consisting of a series of layers, not completely separated from one another like the skins of an onion but merging into one another gradually.

1. The topmost layer, the mineral mass, is related to the interior as an eggshell is to the egg. This layer is called the 'mineral earth'.

2. Under it is a layer called the 'fluid earth'; it consists of a substance to which there is nothing comparable on earth. It is not really like any of the fluids we know. Its substance begins to display certain spiritual qualities. As soon as it is brought into contact with something living, it strives to expel and destroy this life.

3. The 'air earth'. This annuls feelings; for instance, if it is brought into contact with pain, the pain is converted into pleasure, and vice versa. The original form of a feeling is extinguished, rather as the second layer extinguishes life.

4. The 'water earth', or 'form earth' produces in the material realm the effects that occur spiritually in Devachan. There we have the negative pictures of physical things.

5. The 'fruit earth' is full of exuberant energy. Every part of it grows out at once like sponge; it gets larger and larger and is held in place only by the upper layers. It is the underlying life which serves the forms of the layers above it.

6. The 'fire earth' is essentially feeling and will. It is sensitive to pain and would cry out if it were trodden on. It consists entirely of passions.

7. The 'earth mirror' or 'earth reflector' gets its name from the fact that its substance changes all the characteristics of the earth into their opposites.

8. The 'divisive' layer. If with developed power one concentrates on it, something very remarkable appears. For example, a plant held in the midst of this layer appears to be multiplied, and so with everything else. But the essential thing is that this layer disrupts the moral qualities also. Through the power it radiates to the earth's surface, it is responsible for strife and disharmony. In order to overcome this disruptive force, human beings must work together in harmony. That is why this layer was laid down in the earth. The substance of everything evil is prepared and organized there. Quarrelsome people are so constituted that this layer has a particular influence on them. This has been known to everyone who has written out of a true knowledge of the esoteric. Dante in his *Divine Comedy* calls this layer the Cain layer. It was here that the strife between the brothers Cain and Abel had its source.

9. The 'earth core' is the substance through whose

influence black magic arises in the world. The power of spiritual evil comes from this source.

You will see that the human being is related to all the layers, lives under the influence of these layers and has to overcome their powers. When human beings have learnt to radiate life and have trained their breathing so that it promotes life, they will overcome the 'fire earth'. When spiritually they overcome pain through serenity, they overcome the 'air earth'. When concord reigns, the 'divisive' layer is conquered. When white magic triumphs, no evil remains. Human evolution thus implies a transformation of the earth's interior. In the beginning the nature of the earth's body was such as to hold subsequent developments in check. In the end, when human powers have transformed the earth, it will be a spiritualized earth. In this way the human being imparts his own being to the earth.

Evolution moves on from epoch to epoch. However, the future changes recognized by supersensible cognition involve not the earth alone, but the surrounding heavenly bodies in their relation to the earth. The moon will reunite with the earth, for by that time a sufficient number of human souls will have strength enough to make productive use of the reintegrated lunar forces.[118] That will also be a time when, side by side with human souls who have attained this high level of development, others will be living who have turned to a path leading towards evil. These backward souls will have burdened their karma with so much error as to constitute a special group subject to aberration and evil, and bitterly opposed to the progressive community among humankind.

By virtue of their spiritual development, the good part of humanity will then be able to make use of the moon forces and with their help transmute the bad, enabling them to participate in the further evolution of the Earth, albeit as a distinct kingdom. Through this labour of the good part of humanity, the earth—united with the moon—will in due time also become able to reunite with the sun, and with the other planets.

After a cosmic interval[119] the earth will then be transmuted into the Jupiter state. In Jupiter, what we now call the mineral kingdom will no longer exist; the forces of this kingdom will have been changed into plantlike forces. Thus upon Jupiter the vegetable kingdom, though in a different form, will be the lowest. Above it will be the animal kingdom, likewise considerably altered, and then a human kingdom, recognizable as the descendants of the bad part of humanity from earth. Lastly, the descendants of the good humanity will constitute a human kingdom on a higher level. A great part of its work will be to influence and ennoble the souls who have fallen into the other group, so that they may yet gain entrance to it.

In the Venus stage of evolution the plant kingdom too will have disappeared. The lowest will then be the animal kingdom. Above it will be three human kingdoms, differing in degrees of perfection. During the Venus stage the earth will remain united with the sun. From Venus, at a certain stage, a separate celestial body becomes detached. This 'irreclaimable moon' includes all the beings who have persisted in resisting the true course of evolution. It enters upon a line of development such as no words can portray, so utterly unlike is it to anything within the range of the human being's experience on earth. The evolved humanity on the other hand, in a form of existence utterly spiritualized, goes forward into Vulcan evolution.[120]

We see then that the 'knowledge of the Grail' culminates in the highest imaginable ideal of human evolution — the ideal of spiritualization, brought about by the human being's own efforts. This is the ultimate outcome of the harmony achieved in the fifth and sixth epochs of the present age — the harmony between the powers of intelligence and feeling, which the human being has by now acquired, and the true knowledge of the spiritual worlds. What the human being is thus achieving in his own inner life is destined ultimately to become an outer world. Great and sublime are the impressions he receives from his surrounding world. In the aspiration of his mind and spirit as he goes out to meet them, he at first divines and at last clearly recognizes spiritual beings of whom these impressions are the outer garment. His heart responds to the infinite majesty and sublimity of it all. Moreover he begins to know that the experiences and achievements of his own inner life — in intellect, in feeling, in character and strength of purpose — are seeds of a future spiritual world, a world in process of becoming.

We may ask if human freedom is not incompatible with

all this foreknowledge, this predetermination of the cosmic future. But the human being's freedom of action in the earth's future will depend on the predestined cosmic plan no more than will his freedom be impaired by his present resolve in a year's time; he will be as free as his character allows. So too on Jupiter and Venus (again, within the conditions prevailing there) the human being will be free according to the scope and measure of his own inner being. Freedom will depend not on what is predetermined by the cosmic past, but on what the soul has become by its own efforts.

Earth evolution bears within it the outcome of Saturn, Sun and Moon evolutions. In all the processes of nature going on around him, the human being upon earth finds wisdom. Wisdom is present in these processes as the fruit of what was undertaken in the preceding epochs. Earth is the cosmic descendant of Old Moon, which evolved with all its creatures into a 'cosmos of wisdom'. With earth itself, an evolution is beginning whereby a new virtue, a new force, is being added to this wisdom. As a result of earthly evolution, the human being comes to feel himself an independent member of a spiritual world. He owes it to the fact that upon earth the 'I' or ego is engendered in him by the spirits of form.

And in the future, the 'I' of the human being will harmonize with the beings of earth, Jupiter, Venus and Vulcan by virtue of the new force which earthly evolution is implanting in the pristine wisdom. It is the power of love. It has to have its beginning in the human being on earth.

The cosmos of wisdom is thus evolving into a cosmos of love. All that the 'I' of the human being brings to development within him will grow into love. It is the sublime Sun-being of whom we told when describing the evolution of the Christ event, who at his revelation stands forth as the all-embracing prototype of love. The seed of love is thereby planted into the innermost depth of the human being. Thence it shall grow and spread until it fills the whole of cosmic evolution.

Notes

1. Two recent publications highlight the plight of our current situation: *Fast Food Nation* by Eric Schlosser, Penguin 2001; and *The Great Food Gamble* by John Humphrys, Hodder and Stoughton 2001.

2. Steiner stated that 'No one can judge of agriculture who does not derive his judgement from field and forest and the breeding of cattle. All talk of economics which is not derived from the job itself should really cease.' *Agriculture Course*, Lecture 1.

3. First quotation from *Agriculture Course*, Lecture 1. Second quotation from *Agriculture Course*, new edition, Appendix C, pp. 260–1.

4. The agriculture lectures were given at Koberwitz, near Breslau, Silesia from 7 to 16 June 1924.

5. See Anthony Scofield, 'Organic farming: the origin of the name', *Biological Agriculture and Horticulture*, 1986, Vol. 4, pp. 1–5.

6. These were members of the Experimental Circle who worked closely with the School of Spiritual Science at the Goetheanum, Dornach, Switzerland.

7. A selection of these works are listed in the Further Reading section, pp. 231–3.

8. R. Steiner, *At the Gates of Spiritual Science*, Lecture 14, p. 133.

9. Steiner refers both to elemental beings and to nature spirits. These are mostly retarded spirits from a previous epoch. Their spiritual guidance is gradually being withdrawn,

making it important for human beings now to assume this responsibility. See Appendix B, Part 6, p. 254, *Agriculture Course*, 1993 edition.

10   This etheric or life body is an energy system that animates the physical. Ethers are the forces that lie behind material substance.

11   We may refer to the astral body as the body of senses. The word 'astral' has its origin in traditional wisdom.

12   This spiritual member of the human being is otherwise called the 'ego' (Latin = I am) and is the unique individuality that we possess.

13   In this and other respects Steiner's teachings are largely in accordance with Buddhist disciplines.

14   In occult literature, pralaya signifies a spiritual resting period or involution as distinct from a period of evolution (or manvantara). The metamorphosis from spiritual into physical and back to spiritual is called a round or life state. Each round is divided into seven globes or form states: Arupa, Rupa, astral, physical, then back to astral, Rupa and Arupa. Each period of planetary evolution thus passes through 49 metamorphoses.

15   We may visualize this as the combined Moon and Earth after the Sun had departed, hence the term 'Old Moon'.

16   Genesis (literally creation) is the first book of the Judaeo-Christian Bible.

17   See Steiner's remarks about the four elements in Chapter 2. This physical 'warmth' manifestation of humanity is actually a recapitulation of the ancient Saturn evolution during the first or Polarean stage of our earth epoch. Subsequent periods are known as the Hyperborean, Lemurian, Atlantean and Post-Atlantean in which we are at present.

18 The Atlantean period came to a final catastrophic end about 12,000 years ago.

19 The different ethnic groups have had a long period of evolution resulting from the merging of earlier races. It is from the Aryan peoples that modern intellectual and materialistic culture has developed. In our present epoch, the first civilization (sub-race) of the Aryan peoples (12,000–9000 years ago) is known as the ancient Indian.

20 We find therefore that in the Middle East around 9–10,000 years ago moves were made towards tilling the soil, growing crops and domesticating animals. It was the great initiate Zarathustra who gave this impulse.

21 Steiner points out that earlier faculties possessed by Atlantean humanity, which enabled them to breed plants and animals, were transmuted into the Greek sense for aesthetics. *Cosmic Memory*, p. 247.

22 Humanity of the post-Atlantean or present epoch.

23 Steiner states, 'Alcohol is something quite special in the realm of nature. It not only produces a burden for the human organism but becomes a veritable opposing power.' *Nutrition and Stimulants*, p. 159. We can only imagine what he might have said about modern drug abuse.

24 A problem of our time is to visualize space as something other than empty. This question is raised again in Chapter 6, p. 127, where Steiner describes space as spirit-filled and infinitely fertile.

25 This inevitably generates a striving or evolutionary impulse. Similarly, it is to be noted that while each planet has its own rhythmic behaviour, no combinations of planetary rhythms are ever repeated. This means that fresh influences are always possible.

26 These relationships form the basic framework for the current biodynamic farming calendar which has been developed through constant experimentation by Maria Thun over the past 40 years. What Steiner says may appear to contradict current use of this calendar since the moon (or sun) *blocks* rather than *focuses* the influences from each successive zodiacal constellation. However, what we have to consider is that each zodiacal constellation will give plant families their impulse to develop the part of the plant form which is less supported at that time. Plants thus achieve different forms of growth according to specific zodiacal timings of sowing, planting and other essential management.

27 Such ideas have been taken forward very helpfully by Willy Sucher: see Further Reading.

28 Consequently we now see the relationship between states of matter purely in terms of densification or the strengthening of electromagnetic forces within and between adjacent atoms. We think of warmth or heat as the agent by which changes in state are brought about. In reality warmth is the finest of all the 'elements' and therefore can permeate all other conditions of matter.

29 The word 'gas' is of quite recent origin and was coined by van Helmont. He recognized that behind its physical nature a spiritual influence was at work (see Chapter 6, pp. 126–7, for further discussion).

30 See Walter Cloos: Further Reading, p. 232.

31 Further information on the interior of the earth is to be found in *At the Gates of Spiritual Science*, Lecture 14, pp. 129–42.

32 Steiner is of course referring here to the northern hemisphere.

33   Techniques eligible for such investigation would include the various picture-forming methods of quality evaluation, especially chromatographic and crystallization methods (see E.E. Pfeiffer, *Chromatography applied to Quality Testing*, Wyoming, Rhode Island 1984, and *Sensitive Crystallization Processes*, New York 1936).

34   Steiner is not alone in encouraging us to think differently about trees. Viktor Schauberger studied energy flows through trees which appear to corroborate the breathing process already discussed (see C. Coates, *Living Energies*, Gateway Books UK, p. 215).

35   Steiner also states the importance of planetary influences in plants and in our diet, and that 'in his organs man bears within him the images of divine-spiritual beings', *True and False Paths of Spiritual Investigation*, p. 202, London, 1985 (GA 243).

36   On many occasions Steiner refers to the head region of the human being as equivalent to the root system of the plant. There is a parallel between the brain as the seat of our intelligence and the wisdom of the earthbound gnome in the root region of the plant (see Chapter 8). Our present upright situation accords with our orientation when we were plantlike inhabitants of the ancient Sun (see Chapter 1).

37   Steiner controversially likens the processes in the brain with those of the intestines! The point here is that digestion provides raw materials for higher activity than the basic processes of life. Dung is considered as a premature brain deposit. Dunglike matter, he says, 'is transmuted into the noble matter of the brain, there to become a foundation for ego development'. *Agriculture Course*, p. 140.

38   Note that the cow lives in that zone which Steiner has previously described as the 'intestines of the agricultural individuality'. *Agriculture Course*, p. 30.

39   Recent anecdotal evidence of maize yields from northern Ghana appears to confirm this.

40   We note here that Steiner includes other insects with butterflies. Butterflies are clearly a more perfected astral form as well as a source of delight. Elsewhere in the text, reference to 'butterfly' can probably be taken to mean 'flying insects' generally.

41   *Equisetum* introduces silica—a representative of warmth and light to counteract the strong working of the earth-water element. Increased silica content of cells is known to inhibit fungal activity.

42   The oak bark is included among Steiner's six preparations for vitalizing compost (see *Agriculture Course*). This extract is included simply to illustrate his approach to working in a therapeutic way with plants.

43   Occult books give descriptions and pictures of the fundamental entities which compose atoms. A stimulating review of the work of C.W. Leadbeater and A. Besant (published originally as *Occult Chemistry*) appears as Appendix C in *Secrets of the Soil* by P. Tompkins and C. Bird, Viking Arkana, London, 1989. Elsewhere Steiner says that atomic substance is nothing other than congealed electricity and that 'thought' itself is composed of the same substance. *The Temple Legend*, pp. 123, 201–2 (GA 93).

44   Ahriman is the spirit of darkness and materiality which has enabled humanity to gain freedom but which will harden and enslave us if we do not strive for spiritual things. Lucifer is the polar opposite, enticing humanity to

renounce connection with the earth, in which case we would not be able to progress. Our task in life is therefore to try to keep these opposing powers, known in the Bible as Satan and the Devil, in balance, and to take the middle way which Steiner says is the way of Christ.

45 The question of the moon's separation from the earth is discussed in Steiner's book *Cosmic Memory* — see Further Reading, p. 231.

46 We have already encountered this concept in Chapter 4.

47 A recent book concentrates on this theme: *Silica, Lime and Clay* by F. Benesch and K. Wilde, Schaumberg, Illinois 1995.

48 Photosynthesis involves the absorption of carbon dioxide — symbolizing both *form* and *life-bearing* substance. Oxygen and water vapour are by-products of the process.

49 Plant roots take up nitrogen mainly as nitrate, in other words where nitrogen is combined with oxygen. This is a simple illustration of nitrogen guiding the life principle (oxygen) to the structures (in the plant) provided by the carbon.

50 Steiner actually used here the expression 'Universal All' which will be better understood after consideration of Chapter 6.

51 This statement of the role of hydrogen is very reminiscent of Steiner's remarks about birds and insects in the spiritualization of matter. He makes no link between them, but experience with Steiner's work would suggest that he is looking at the same phenomenon from different vantage points. (See also Chapter 6, p. 126.)

52 Steiner is here referring to the biodynamic preparations — see Chapter 7 for some examples or the Further Reading list for full details.

53   This is a most important passage. Lower kingdoms support those above them. In this case the mineral supports the plant or human being. When the mineral substance—in this case nitrogen—enters a living organism (or the soil) it becomes alive. In other words, its forces are released into the etheric body of the organism and it becomes part of a process instead of remaining as a discrete substance. Steiner is saying that the potential value of the nitrogen (but it could be any other substance) released into the plant depends on its previous involvement with a living rather than purely mineral or synthetic process.

54   The implication of these remarks is that without a living soil the life ether drawn from the outer planets will be weakened. Living soil is required constantly to generate humus, which is effectively organic matter returned to the mineral realm. In this form, previously living chemical structures combine with clay minerals providing a focus for crystallizing forces from the cosmos. This allows a better understanding of Steiner's reference to forces 'penetrating' earthly substance.

55   All living material yields an *etheric* or *living* quality while the *astral* element arises from the additional complexity of animal life over plants. The decomposing remains of animals or their dung will therefore contain what Steiner refers to as astrality, which amounts to an enhanced *sensitivity to cosmic influences*.

56   These remarks are not so dated as might appear. Readers may be aware of the existence of what are called effective micro-organisms or EM. While the decomposition of very specialized or nutritionally unbalanced materials may require appropriate 'starter' organisms, all normal com-

posting can be carried out without any such intervention. For most purposes there is no need to accelerate normal decomposition rates and to do so incurs risks. The importation of organisms is arguably against the principles of the farm organism as discussed in Chapter 4.

57   While lime (or dolomite) is commonly used in the compost-making process, its role can be substituted by ash provided this is from uncontaminated materials.

58   These remarks are of particular relevance for the production of compost in heaps or windows. They also provide a further justification for the development of raised beds for intensive cropping.

59   It is apparent here that Steiner is not talking about manure or compost as a fertilizer material but as activating the earth element around the plant and, other things being equal, raising the potential of the soil to provide beneficial nutrition.

60   There is indeed a continuum from the plant root to the humus and minerals in the soil at large. In practice the root is prolonged by fungal mycorrhizae and surrounded by countless types of bacteria, so there is no real meaning in separating soil from plant.

61   Steiner refers here to the biodynamic compost preparations—see Chapter 7, pp. 134–41, and Further Reading, pp. 231–33.

62   The implication here is of micro-nutrient (or trace element) deficiencies.

63   But we should note that the soil needs to be endowed with humus in order for these substances to be 'radiated in' effectively. This suggests that organic management generates true sustainability at least as regards certain elements.

64   Heavier substances cannot escape the earth. Hydrogen can, while the proton, as its essence, is present in all larger elements. This, and the clear evidence of a memory effect in water, may help to explain how hydrogen performs this cosmic role. However, it is water vapour that holds the key to this mystery. It is this, not hydrogen as such, which leaves when organisms die. It is in the upper atmosphere that earthly molecules are subject to breakdown. Here, water breaks down to hydrogen and monatomic oxygen.

65   The reader should also consult *Nature Spirits*, Lecture 7, pp. 115–16.

66   Steiner is here referring especially to cow dung with forces concentrated in it as described in the section 'The cow, her horns and manure' of Chapter 4, pp. 80–4.

67   The main purpose of alternately creating and destroying vortices is to ensure that the essence of the preparation has passed into (or has penetrated) the water. Other influences on the liquid such as cosmic forces and effects derived from the person stirring are also to be considered. The vortex is one of water's most frequently occurring forms and has a generally enlivening effect upon it. See, for example, T. Schwenk, *Sensitive Chaos*, London 1996; A. Hall, *Water, Electricity and Health*, Hawthorn Press 1997.

68   This so-called 'horn manure' is sprinkled or sprayed onto the soil with coarse drops at or before sowing or planting. The operation should be carried out in the evening.

69   The season for burying the manure or silica horn is determined by the low or high sun period of the year, not on other seasonal weather characteristics. This connects with the earth's breathing process as discussed on pp. 60–7. In the case of the 'horn silica', spraying as a fine mist over leaf

surfaces should be done in the early morning, preferably around sunrise. In the weeks before harvesting, spraying is, however, done in the afternoon or evening.

70 The word 'manure' is here taken to include both fresh animal excrement or farmyard manure, as well as all other animal and vegetable residues involved in a composting process.

71 With the compost-vitalizing preparations we are involved with different planetary influences that govern the processes connected with certain chemical elements. Yarrow, for example, was known traditionally as Venus' eyebrow. Several compost preparations involve the use of an animal organ, which raises the energy of the preparation to the more potent and sensitive astral level.

72 In this statement there could be no better illustration of the method by which earthly substance is vitalized by the activated compost.

73 This is a very interesting reference to the concept of element 'isotopes' a number of years before these were actually recognized.

74 Steiner's use of 'silicic acid' can be treated broadly to include the element silicon and the oxide, silica, but also any amphoteric substance that can form an acid or a base, such as aluminium (itself a major constituent of silicate minerals).

75 In this passage Steiner has been referring to biologically induced transmutations of elements. Although currently disputed, this was known and experienced by medieval alchemists yet is unlikely to have been exploited for material gain. Once again, organic soil management is said to be vital for the achievement of such processes. As soil is

such a complex material, current scientific experimental design would appear to be incapable of verifying or disproving such ideas. For further reference see C.L. Kervran, *Biological Transmutations*, Crosby Lockwood, 1971; *Alchemy: the Evolution of the Mysteries*, selections from the work of Rudolf Steiner, Sophia Books, 2001.

76   Here, as with the earlier description of the effect of the biodynamic preparations, we are dealing not with physical substance but with forces or effects that are radiative.

77   Here, reference is made to homoeopathic potentization where increasing dilution brings about intensifications of energy in a rhythmic manner according to the substance. In this case the 8th potency has been shown to be effective. See M. Thun, *Gardening for Life*, Hawthorn Press, 1999.

78   The high or 'superior' conjunction here recommended is when Venus is on the far side of the sun. While this may be optimal it greatly limits the time when the preparation can be made. The method will in practice work so long as Venus is passing through Scorpio, which it does during the month of November.

79   These elemental beings will be introduced in the next section.

80   According to Steiner, the elemental world is one which can only be perceived by what he called *Imagination*. One can also call the elemental world the imaginative world. (Bern, 9 November 1916 — GA 168. See also *Knowledge of the Higher Worlds*.)

81   St John's time is the summer solstice, which occurs in late June. Michaelmas is the autumnal equinox, which occurs in late September. The seasons are of course reversed for the southern hemisphere.

82 Hagemann states that 'One can look upon higher elemental beings as willing helpers of the creative hierarchical beings, who can move freely in the cosmos until they sacrifice themselves and create things in the four nature kingdoms under the direction of hierarchical beings. Elemental beings have the important task of creating the etheric bodies of all living organisms on earth.' *World Ether*, p. 11.

83 Elemental beings in many cases are those beings which fell behind in their evolution in previous epochs. They are therefore not fitted to take up physical bodies at the present time and have tasks that largely support other beings. Elemental beings can also arise from human actions, and in the case of our weaknesses they can subsequently prove a hindrance to our progress.

84 Glimpses of the elemental world survived into the sixteenth and seventeenth centuries in Europe, as shown by the works of such figures as Shakespeare and Paracelsus.

85 Imagination, Inspiration and Intuition are three perceptive faculties developed on the anthroposophical path of knowledge. Rudolf Steiner described these and ways of achieving them on many occasions. See his *Occult Science. An Outline*, Rudolf Steiner Press, London 1979; a clear exposition is also given in his *Fruits of Anthroposophy*, Rudolf Steiner Press, London 1986.

86 See Ariel's Song in *The Tempest* by William Shakespeare: 'Where the bee sucks, there suck I . . .'

87 It is perhaps surprising that Steiner makes only one reference to 'nature spirits' in his *Agriculture Course*. Of yarrow he says, 'In no other plant do the nature spirits attain such perfection in the use of sulphur' (pp. 91–2).

88 Steiner explains that gnomes live with a constant fear of

becoming amphibians (that is if they fall from their spiritual striving into earthly matter) while undines have a rather similar anxiety about becoming fishes (falling into the physical watery element).

89   Here Steiner has used the example of the life cycle of blue-green algae and their phosphorescence. We must imagine that this is one of many such pictures applying to the natural world.

90   The terms 'elemental being' and 'nature spirit' tend to be used interchangeably. It is important to realize that there are innumerable types of such entities and that in nature there is a hierarchy. A range of elementals connect with the human being. See for example Lectures 3–5 in *Nature Spirits* and B. Lievegoed, *Man on the Threshold*, Hawthorn Press, Stroud 1985, pp. 85–8.

91   Steiner stated: 'It is important to realize that in eating one should develop a vivid relationship to the various kinds of food. For what one experiences in tasting is the living relationship of the macrocosm to the microcosm, an inter-relationship carried on subconsciously in the astral body which penetrates all organs.' *Mirror Images and Realities*, December 1914, GA 156.

92   Hagemann has calculated that 20–35g of cosmic nourishment are needed daily in order to replace bodily substances which are lost (*World Ether*, p. 88).

93   K. König says that as we inhale air, warmth is 'exhaled' into our bodies. This carries light, sound and life (ethers), which meet in the lymph. This cosmic stream as it descends leaves light behind in our head and sound in our rhythmic system. The life goes right down into physical substance and this is what really fills and nourishes us. The life ether is

what takes hold of the carbon passed over from our digestion. The organs that regulate the rising earthly stream and the descending cosmic stream are the endocrine glands. (*Earth and Man*, Biodynamic Literature, Wyoming, Rhode Island, USA 1982.)

94   This connects in a most wonderful way with all that has been said in earlier chapters, on our evolution, the nature of the elements and the tasks of the elemental beings.

95   It is the *forces* we derive from each part of the plant which connect with the different parts of our body. Thus, while green leaves support our chest and rhythmic system they give us the capacity to form our own fats through interaction with the cosmic stream.

96   These various references to cooking cause us to consider what revolutionary changes occurred when earlier humanity first began to cook their food. Equally, we can pause to consider the consequences of the various ways in which our food is cooked or otherwise prepared at the present time.

97   For a more comprehensive discussion of nutrition from a similar perspective, the reader is directed to *Foodwise* by Wendy E. Cook — see Further Reading, p. 232.

98   While Steiner goes out of his way to allow for meat eating, he is here hinting at the fact that for those engaged on a path of spiritual development or who are calling upon spiritual faculties there really is no substitute for a largely vegetarian diet.

99   This underlines the whole philosophy of organic and biodynamic agriculture. Evidence of the superior quality of organic and biodynamic produce can be examined in two recent publications: V. Worthington, *Nutrition and Biody-*

namics (Kimberton, USA) 1999; *Organic Farming, Food Quality and Human Health,* Soil Association (UK), 2001.

100 For an interpretation of these divisions, see for example Steiner, *Harmony of the Creative Word,* especially Lectures 1–3.

101 This is directly connected to the foregoing remarks about our digestion.

102 Besides our concern for cattle let us also consider the natural needs of poultry to scratch in the soil, for a perch above ground at night and enough space to move about. The pig requires to root about in the soil and despite its reputation it will naturally organize its own hygiene better than when kept on concrete. Denial of dignified conditions for animals creates stress, ill-health and inevitably a lower quality of food for human beings.

103 It is of interest to note that this gesture carries the signature of silica in the plant world.

104 Many animal breeds today, originating in one area, have become widespread. We have therefore to consider ways of helping the animals to connect more fully with the earth and landscape of each different location, thus fulfilling an essential aspect of the farm individuality.

105 According to Steiner (*Agriculture Course,* p. 72), 'Anyone who wishes to understand foot-and-mouth disease — that is, the action of the periphery on the digestive tract — must clearly perceive this relationship. Our remedy for foot-and-mouth disease is founded on this perception.' The actual remedy was originally published in J. Werr, *Animal Husbandry and Animal Medicine in the Framework of Bio-Dynamic Agriculture,* Stuttgart, 1953. A situation potentially provoking this disease is to force the bovine organism to greater production without consideration of the necessary

forces radiating back into the digestive system (see section 'Animals and the farm individuality' in Chapter 4).

106 These remarks, of direct relevance to the recent history of BSE, were made in a lecture by Rudolf Steiner on 13 January 1923 (*From Comets to Cocaine*, pp. 226–8).

107 These terms refer to people who have had access to knowledge from spiritual sources. They may have gained this from their own inner development or from spiritual leaders or initiates.

108 Faculties may indeed slumber in human beings but 'In times when there were no electrical currents, when the air was not swarming with electrical influences, it was easier to be human. For this reason it is necessary to expend much stronger spiritual capacities than was necessary a century ago.' Steiner's reaction is not to banish all technical achievements but he urges that 'modern human beings need the access to the spirit that spiritual science provides, so that through this experience they can become stronger in relation to the forces that accompany modern culture. R. Steiner, lecture of 11 July 1923 in *Die menschliche Seele in ihrem Zusammenhang mit göttlich-geistigen Individualitäten* (GA 224).

109 Further information on methods of meditation is to be found in Steiner's *Knowledge of the Higher Worlds* and *Occult Science*. An important attitude of mind arises from realizing that the physical world, the astral or world of soul, and the devachanic or world of spirit are in fact not spatially separate but interpenetrate. 'When the senses of the soul are opened, the new world with its new characteristics and new beings emerges. In proportion as a person acquires new senses, so are new phenomena revealed to him.' R. Steiner, *At the Gates of Spiritual Science*, pp. 18–19.

110   On a number of occasions in the *Agriculture Course* Steiner mentions the importance of developing a personal relationship towards what one does, for example (p. 69), 'We must know how to gain a kind of personal relationship to all things that concern our farming work and above all a personal relationship to the manure, especially to the task of working with the manure.' This special relationship can be seen as deriving partly from a deepened understanding of the material one is creating or working with, and partly from a state of mind which is concentrated on the activity in a meditative way and is not distracted by other preoccupations.

111   The practice of using mantras or chanting to control pests and animal predation of crops is still employed with effect in certain parts of the East but, significantly, only by people of high moral standing.

112   In other words we must reunite ourselves spiritually with the rhythms of the earth; thereby we strengthen links with helpful elemental beings as well as with higher spiritual powers.

113   Random, or perhaps cyclical, are other ways in which natural events have been described.

114   Hagemann in *World Ether* (p. 44) gives further examples of the need for human beings to take responsibility for elemental beings.

115   Rudolf Steiner in conversation with Kurt Walther, Aug. 12, 1920 (See Sources).

116   We should recall the treatment of this subject in Chapter 2 and its further elaboration in Chapter 6.

117   In fact, this is one respect in which science has made progress since Steiner's time. Few scientists today would be so unimaginative.

118 Steiner is at this point talking about the later stages of the Earth evolutionary period.

119 Steiner is here referring to a *pralaya* or period in an entirely spiritual condition.

120 See also *Cosmic Memory*, Chapter 13, 'The Earth and its Future', pp. 164–73.

Sources

A special note on sources

References to the *Agriculture Course* refer to the edition of 1958 (now out of print) where the English translation was by George Adams. *Agriculture Course* New Edition refers to the 1993 volume translated by Catherine Creeger and Malcolm Gardner — see Further Reading, p. 231.

1. The Evolving Human Being

The contemporary human being
At the Gates of Spiritual Science, London 1986, pp. 11–16 (GA 95)

Former evolutionary stages
Cosmic Memory, New York 1987, pp. 154–5
At the Gates of Spiritual Science, pp. 81–5
Occult Science, London 1963, p. 139 (GA 13)
Genesis, London 1959, pp. 108–10 (GA 122)

The emergence of modern consciousness
Cosmic Memory, p. 42
Egyptian Myths and Mysteries, New York 1971, p. 29 (GA 106)
At the Gates of Spiritual Science, pp. 98–100
Egyptian Myths and Mysteries, pp. 94, 96–7, 99
Man and the World of Stars, London 1963, pp. 113–14 (GA 219)
Lucifer and Ahriman, New York 1993, pp. 8–9 (GA 191/193)

The significance of changes in nutrition
Foundations of Esotericism, London 1982, pp. 242–7 (GA 93a)
Nutrition and Stimulants, Kimberton 1991, pp. 65–6, 163 (GA 354)

2. Cosmos as the Source of Life

Stars and the significance of the zodiac
Lucifer and Ahriman, p. 73
Mystery of the Universe, London 2001, pp. 58–9 (GA 201)
Agriculture Course, L6 p. 115 (GA 327)
Harmony of the Creative Word, London 2001, p. 22 (GA 230)
Mystery of the Universe, pp. 83–4
From Beetroot to Buddhism, London 1999, pp. 206–8 (GA 353)

The Sun and its planetary relationships
Mystery of the Universe, pp. 48–9
Warmth Course, New York 1988, p. 9 (GA 321)
Astronomy Course, Lecture 18 (Typescript 3 pp) (GA 323)
Mystery of the Universe, pp. 52–3, 56

Elementary conditions and spiritual beings
Genesis, pp. 76–9

The nature of the four primal elements
Warmth Course, pp. 28–9, 68–9, 78–9

3. Plants and the Living Earth

Plants, minerals and creation
Genesis, pp. 70–1
The Spirit in the Realm of Plants, New York 1984, pp. 8–10

The plant world between earth and sun
The Spirit in the Realm of Plants, pp. 8–9

The World of the Senses and the World of the Spirit, Vancouver 1979, pp. 80–1 (GA 134)
The Spirit in the Realm of Plants, pp. 18, 23–4, 27

Earth's seasonal and diurnal breathing processes
The Cycle of the Year as Breathing Process of the Earth, New York 1984, pp. 1–3, 6–11 (GA 223)
Man and the World of Stars, pp. 118–19
Agriculture Course, L2 pp. 33–4
Warmth Course, pp. 88–90

Trees and the astral environment of plants
Cosmic Workings in Earth and Man, London 1952, pp. 65–9
Agriculture Course, pp. 126–9
Mirror Images and Realities, Lecture 2, from 4 lectures, Dornach, 12–20 December 1914. Translated typescript, pp. 7–8 (GA 156)

4. Farms and the Realms of Nature

Animals and the farm individuality
Agriculture Course, L2 pp. 29–31, 39–40, 41, L7 p. 132, L8 pp. 140–1

The cow, her horns and manure
Harmony of the Creative Word, pp. 10, 25–6
Agriculture Course, L4 pp. 72–3

The mission of birds and insects
Agriculture Course, L7 pp. 128–30
Bees, New York 1998, p. 20 (GA 348/351)
Harmony of the Creative Word, pp. 68–70, 73–4

Fungi and plant disease
Agriculture Course, L5 pp. 96–7, L6 pp. 116–18, L7 pp. 132–3

5. Bringing the Chemical Elements to Life

The nature of the atom
Warmth Course, p. 171
Karma of Materialism, New York 1985, pp. 33–5 (GA 176)

Planetary influences on earthly life
Agriculture Course, L1 p. 23
Introducing Anthroposophical Medicine, New York 1999, pp. 84–6
(GA 312)
Agriculture Course, L2 pp. 36–7, L6 pp. 109–10

Silica, lime and clay
Agriculture Course, L1 pp. 23–5, L2 pp. 31–2, L3 p. 55

The elements of organic substance
Agriculture Course, L3 pp. 42–4, 45–50, 52–3, 55

6. Soil and the World of Spirit

Nurturing the life of the soil
Agriculture Course, L5 p. 87–8
Agriculture Course, New Edition, pp. 9–10, 136–7
Agriculture Course, L4 pp. 68–9, 70, 70–71, 88, L5 pp. 88–90

The resonance of chaos and cosmos
Agriculture Course, L2 pp. 34–6, L3 p. 52
On Chaos and Cosmos, lecture, Berlin, 19 October 1907 (GA 284)

7. Supporting and Regulating Life Processes

Field sprays to invigorate soil and plant
Agriculture Course, L4 pp. 73–5

Vitalizing solid or liquid organic fertilizers
Agriculture Course, L5 pp. 90–96, 98–100

Suppressing the growth of weeds
Agriculture Course, L6 pp. 110–11, 116

Regulating the abundance of pests
Agriculture Course, L6 pp. 112–15

8. Spirits of the Elements

Elementals as the manifestation of cosmic forces
Harmony of the Creative Word, p. 127
The Cycle of the Year as Breathing Process of the Earth, pp. 39–41
World Ether (Steiner, compiled by E. Hagemann and containing additional sources), New York 1993, pp. 11–12, 14

Elemental beings of the plant kingdom
Harmony of the Creative Word, pp. 109–11, 113–24, 126

Elementals as gatherers of substance
Harmony of the Creative Word, pp. 146–50

9. Nutrition and Vitality

New concepts in nutrition
World Ether, pp. 86–7
Harmony of the Creative Word, p. 81

The plant and the digestive process
Two Lectures to Workmen, New York 1987, pp. 5–23 (also reproduced in *Nutrition and Stimulants,* Chapters 17 and 18) (GA 354)

The nutrition and health of animals
Agriculture Course, L8 pp. 136–9, 141–3, 144, 145–7

Bees, pp. 71–2
From Comets to Cocaine, London 2000, pp. 226–8 (GA 348)

10. Responsibility for the Future

The inner challenge for the human being
Knowledge of the Higher Worlds: How is it achieved? London 1976,
pp. 19, 21, 23–7, 29–31 (GA 10)

Human influence on nature's processes
Agriculture Course, First Discussion, pp. 83–4
Lucifer and Ahriman, pp. 74–6
Man and the World of Stars, Lecture 12, pp. 183–4

Recognizing the needs of spiritual beings
Agriculture Course, New Edition, Appendix B, pp. 254–5
Nature Spirits, London 1995, pp. 51–2
How does one bring reality of being into the world of ideas? Mirror images and realities, Lecture 3, Typescript, pp. 18–19 (GA 156)

The long-term goal of humanity
At the Gates of Spiritual Science, London 1986, pp. 137–40 (GA 95)
Occult Science – An Outline, London 1969, pp. 308–11 (GA 13)

Note on Rudolf Steiner's lectures
Readers wishing to search more thoroughly through Steiner's agriculturally related work in German may be interested to know of the intensively researched publication by Thomas van Elsen, *Gesichtspunkte für ökologische Leitbilder des Biologisch-Dynamischen Landbaus im Vortragswerk Rudolf Steiners,* Witzenhausen 1996 (In der langen Grund 2, 37217 Witzenhausen, Germany).

Further Reading

By Rudolf Steiner

The Cycle of the Year as Breathing Process of the Earth, Hudson, New York 1984 (GA 223)

Nature Spirits, London 1995

An Outline of Esoteric Science, Great Barrington, MA, 1997 (earlier editions published as *Occult Science*) (GA 13)

Mystery of the Universe – The Human Being, Image of Creation, London 2001 (originally published as *Man: Hieroglyph of the Universe*) (GA 201)

Harmony of the Creative Word – The Human Being and the Elemental, Animal, Plant and Mineral Kingdoms, London 2001 (originally published as *Man as Symphony of the Creative Word*) (GA 230)

Bees, Hudson, New York, 1998 (GA 348/351)

Nutrition and Stimulants, Kimberton, PA, 1991. Lectures and extracts compiled and translated by K. Castellitz and B. Saunders-Davies

Cosmic Memory – Prehistory of Earth and Man, Blauvelt, New York, 1987 (GA 11)

Spiritual Foundations for the Renewal of Agriculture, Kimberton, PA, 1993 (the most recent edition of the *Agriculture Course* given in 1924)

Founding a Science of the Spirit, London 1999 (originally published as *At the Gates of Spiritual Science*) (GA 95)

Introducing Anthroposophical Medicine, Hudson, New York, 1999 (GA 312)

The Spirit in the Realm of Plants, Spring Valley, New York, 1984

Understanding the Human Being – Selected writings of Rudolf Steiner, Bristol 1993. Edited by Richard Seddon

World Ether – Elemental Beings – Kingdoms of Nature, Spring Valley, New York, 1993. Texts from Rudolf Steiner's spiritual science compiled and with a commentary by Ernst Hagemann

'Answers to Questions', a series of 7 volumes, London 1999–2002: *From Beetroot to Buddhism, From Mammoths to Mediums, From Limestone to Lucifer, From Elephants to Einstein, From Comets to Cocaine, From Crystals to Crocodiles, From Sunspots to Strawberries.*

By other authors

George Adams and Olive Whicher, *The Plant between Sun and Earth,* Stourbridge 1952

Walter Cloos, *The Living Earth – The Organic Origin of Rocks and Minerals,* 1977

Wendy E. Cook, *Foodwise: understanding what we eat and how it affects us – the story of human nutrition,* Forest Row 2003

Lawrence Edwards, *The Vortex of Life – Nature's Patterns in Space and Time,* Edinburgh 1993

Adalbert Graf von Keyserlingk, *The Birth of a New Agriculture – Koberwitz 1924,* London 1999

Herbert Koepf, *The Biodynamic Farm – Agriculture in the Service of the Earth and Humanity,* Hudson, New York, 1989

Ehrenfried Pfeiffer, *Soil Fertility, Renewal and Preservation – Biodynamic Farming and Gardening,* East Grinstead 1983

Gita Henderson (editor), *Biodynamic Perspectives: Farming and Gardening,* Auckland 2001

Jules Pretty, *Agri-Culture: Reconnecting People, Land and Nature*, London 2002

Friedrich Sattler and Eckard von Wistinghausen, *Biodynamic Farming Practice*, Stourbridge 1992

Willy Schilthuis, *Biodynamic Agriculture*, Edinburgh 1994

Wolf Storl, *Culture and Horticulture – A Philosophy of Gardening*, Wyoming, RI, 1979

Theodor and Wolfram Schwenk, *Water – the Element of Life*, Hudson, New York, 1989

Willi Sucher, *The Living Universe and the New Millennium*, Stourbridge 1997. Lectures compiled by Hazel Straker

Maria Thun, *Gardening for Life – The Biodynamic Way*, Stroud 1999

Note Regarding Rudolf Steiner's Lectures

The lectures and addresses contained in this volume have been translated from the German, which is based on stenographic and other recorded texts that were in most cases never seen or revised by the lecturer. Hence, due to human errors in hearing and transcription, they may contain mistakes and faulty passages. Every effort has been made to ensure that this is not the case. Some of the lectures were given to audiences more familiar with anthroposophy; these are the so-called 'private' or 'members' lectures. Other lectures, like the written works, were intended for the general public. The difference between these, as Rudolf Steiner indicates in his *Autobiography*, is twofold. On the one hand, the members' lectures take for granted a background in and commitment to anthroposophy; in the public lectures this was not the case. At the same time, the members' lectures address the concerns and dilemmas of the members, while the public work speaks directly out of Steiner's own understanding of universal needs. Nevertheless, as Rudolf Steiner stresses: 'Nothing was ever said that was not solely the result of my direct experience of the growing content of anthroposophy. There was never any question of concessions to the prejudices and preferences of the members. Whoever reads these privately printed lectures can take them to represent anthroposophy in the fullest sense. Thus it was possible without hesitation—when the complaints in this direction became too persistent—to depart from the custom of circulating this material "For members only". But it must be borne in mind that faulty passages do occur in these reports not revised by myself.' Earlier in the same chapter, he states: 'Had I been able to correct them [the private lectures], the restriction *for members only* would have been unnecessary from the beginning.'

The original German editions on which this text is based were published by Rudolf Steiner Verlag, Dornach, Switzerland in the collected edition (*Gesamtausgabe*, 'GA') of Rudolf Steiner's work. All publications are edited by the Rudolf Steiner Nachlassverwaltung (estate), which wholly owns both Rudolf Steiner Verlag and the Rudolf Steiner Archive. The organization relies solely on donations to continue its activity.

For further information please contact:

Rudolf Steiner Archiv
Postfach 135
CH-4143 Dornach

or:

www.rudolf-steiner.com

Rudolf Steiner

ARCHITECTURE
An Introductory Reader

Compiled with an introduction, commentary and notes by
Andrew Beard

The origins and nature of architecture
The formative influence of architectural forms
The history of architecture in the light of mankind's spiritual
  evolution
A new architecture as a means of uniting with spiritual forces
Art and architecture as manifestations of spiritual realities
Metamorphosis in architecture
Aspects of a new architecture
Rudolf Steiner on the first Goetheanum building
The second Goetheanum building
The architecture of a community in Dornach
The temple is the human being
The restoration of the lost temple

ISBN 1 85584 123 1

Rudolf Steiner

ART
An Introductory Reader

Compiled with an introduction, commentary and notes by
Anne Stockton

The being of the arts
Goethe as the founder of a new science of aesthetics
Technology and art
At the turn of each new millennium
The task of modern art and architecture
The living walls
The glass windows
Colour on the walls
Form—moving the circle
The seven planetary capitals of the first Goetheanum
The model and the statue 'The Representative of Man'
Colour and faces
Physiognomies

ISBN 1 85584 138 X

Rudolf Steiner

EDUCATION
An Introductory Reader

Compiled with an introduction, commentary and notes by
Christopher Clouder

A social basis for education
The spirit of the Waldorf school
Educational methods based on anthroposophy
The child at play
Teaching from a foundation of spiritual insight and education in
   the light of spiritual science
The adolescent after the fourteenth year
Science, art, religion and morality
The spiritual grounds of education
The role of caring in education
The roots of education and the kingdom of childhood
Address at a parents' evening
Education in the wider social context

ISBN 1 85584 118 5

Rudolf Steiner

MEDICINE
An Introductory Reader

Compiled with an introduction, commentary and notes by
Dr Andrew Maendl

Understanding man's true nature as a basis for medical practice
The science of knowing
The mission of reverence
The four temperaments
The bridge between universal spirituality and the physical
The constellation of the supersensible bodies
The invisible human within us: the pathology underlying
therapy
Cancer and mistletoe, and aspects of psychiatry
Case history questions: diagnosis and therapy
Anthroposophical medicine in practice: three case histories

ISBN 1 85584 133 9

Rudolf Steiner

RELIGION
An Introductory Reader

Compiled with an introduction, commentary and notes by
Andrew Welburn

Mysticism and beyond: the importance of prayer
The meaning of sin and grace
Rediscovering the Bible
What is true communion?
Rediscovering the festivals and the life of the earth
Finding one's destiny: walking with Christ
The significance of religion in life and death
Christ's second coming: the truth for our time
Universal religion: the meaning of love

ISBN 1 85584 128 2

Rudolf Steiner

SCIENCE
An Introductory Reader

Compiled with an introduction, commentary and notes by
Howard Smith

From pre-science to science
The origin of mathematics
The roots of physics and chemistry, and the urge to experiment
Are there limits to what science can know?
Understanding organisms: Goethe's method
The quest for archetypal phenomena
Light, darkness and colour
The rediscovery of the elements
What is warmth?
The scale of nature
The working of the ethers in the physical
Sub-nature; What are atoms?
Natural science and spiritual science

ISBN 1 85584 108 8

Rudolf Steiner

SOCIAL AND POLITICAL SCIENCE
An Introductory Reader

Compiled with an introduction, commentary and notes by
Stephen E. Usher

Psychological cognition
The social question
The social question and theosophy
Memoranda of 1917
The metamorphosis of intelligence
Culture, law and economy
Central Europe between East and West

ISBN 1 85584 103 7